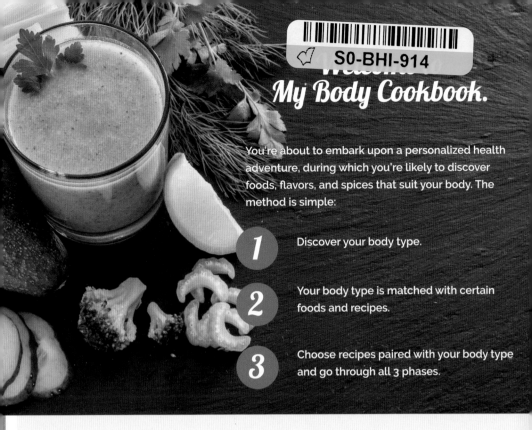

My Body Cookbook.

You're about to embark upon a personalized health adventure, during which you're likely to discover foods, flavors, and spices that suit your body. The method is simple:

1 Discover your body type.

2 Your body type is matched with certain foods and recipes.

3 Choose recipes paired with your body type and go through all 3 phases.

*NOTE: We're not going to ask you to count a single calorie. In fact, you get to eat as much as you want (within reason) every single day, so long as you take your time while you eat and stick to the recipes in this guide. Food is energy, and optimal eating is about finding the match for your body that satisfies you and your every craving.

THE THREE PHASES OF MY BODY COOKBOOK ARE:

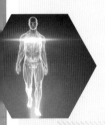

Detox phase:
This is the period of time when the intention is to provide rest and an opportunity for regeneration for your most active body system(s) based upon your body type.

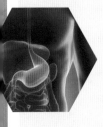

Transition phase:
Before returning to a normal diet, it's important to transition how you eat, in order to restore proper balance of stomach acid, digestive enzymes, and autonomic homeostasis -- or the balance of your nervous system's interpretation of fight or flight vs rest and digest -- since digestion of solid foods takes longer and requires more metabolic effort.

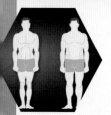

Lifestyle phase: This is the period of time when the intention is to provide rest and an opportunity for regeneration for your body system(s) most active, based upon your body type.

Super simple, right? Choose your body type and then select your favorite recipes from each section for the designated amount of time. If you think you didn't choose the right body type, simply go back to the beginning and start again.

If you're ready to get started, please go to page:

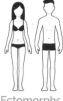

Ectomorphs
(page 16)

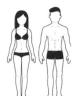

Mesomorphs
(page 17)

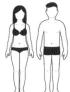

Endomorphs
(page 18)

Of course moving your body also matters and for each body type the movements and exercises need to be a bit different. That's why personalized workouts are so important. If you'd like to be able to build some personalized workouts for free, please visit: http://CreateMyWorkout.com/ VIP and we'll gladly give you a free trial in *Create My Workout* + we'll even discount your future membership as a thank you for trusting us with My Body Cookbook.

You can also access your 100% free workouts by clicking the link below

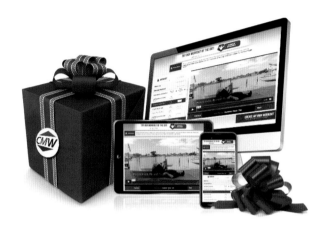

Discounted Doctor-Designed Workouts
Personalized For You
https://CreateMyWorkout.com/free-workouts

TIME TO DETOX

THE SCIENCE OF MY BODY COOKBOOK:

We are meant to eat differently, depending upon our shape and size, ancestry, activity level, prior choices, mood/feeling/emotions, health status, and genetic expression on a minute-to-minute basis. To say there is a single solution for eating that is appropriate for everyone is a big and bold lie. Food simply doesn't work that way.

If I ask you a couple of questions, this might start to make a lot more sense:

> *Is there any arguing that a bear is meant to eat more food than a human?*
>
> *And does it make sense that a lion eats meat, and that a small fish eat algae?*

Sure, some animals -- like deer -- are meant to eat more or less the same diet, regardless of shape or size. However, when we consider animals that have a larger variety of shapes and sizes -- like the distinction between chimpanzees, gorillas, orangutans, and baboons -- it starts to become clear that shape, size, and natural living environment play a huge role in how each of these monkeys is meant to eat.

And we know this to be true across different whale species, too. For example, some orcas (killer whales) only eat salmon, and others eat marine mammals like sharks, seals, etc. This is based upon where they live, where they migrate (what their habits are), food availability, and socialization with the 'pod' (group) of orcas with whom they live. Of course, over time the orcas' diet changes the regulation and secretion of enzymes in their bodies, how they digest, and in turn, which foods they should eat.

Naturally, the same thing is true for humans. Depending upon how petite -- or large -- you are, you require different foods.

Depending upon the choices you make, you require different foods.

Depending upon where you live, weather conditions, socialization, your state of mind, and amount of time you have to digest, you require different foods.

Think about it... this is super simple, when you step away from all the bogus, generalized health information you keep hearing about the 'best' way to lose weight, eat right, or look great. It's all about some 'method' you follow that forces you to restrict yourself from eating your "favorite" foods.

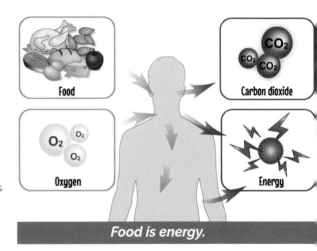

Food

Oxygen

Carbon dioxide

Energy

Food is energy.

Almost every single diet book out there is based upon allowance or restriction of your favorite foods; in other words, they are intentionally -- or inadvertently -- reinforcing emotional eating habits. And, the whole point of 'how' to eat to become healthy gets missed.

Please allow me to say this clearly: you are meant to see food as an energy source. Food is not intended to be chosen simply on flavor, since many of our favorite "foods" are not 'food', at all.

If you showed a vanilla cream donut to a deer, it might want a bite of it, but I think we can all agree that donuts are not 'food' for a deer. Similarly, they're not food for you either. They don't come from nature, they're not seasonal, and you don't naturally have the composition to adequately digest real food when you poison -- or block up -- your system with so-called foods that are not really foods, at all.

BODY AGING THROUGH FOOD, ENVIRONMENT, AND STRESS:

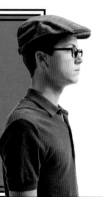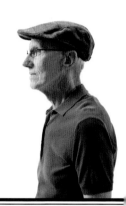

"It's distinctly possible your body's organs are aging faster than you are, biologically speaking. In other words, your 'physiological age is the rate at which your body is aging vs your 'biological' age is your chronological age, in terms of days, weeks, months, and years."

And depending upon the choices you make, how much each of your systems is under stress, and how often you take the time to de-stress priority organs for your body, you may find that your body's organs are aging much slower than expected, or much faster. Some easy examples to understand how environment affects body organ health include:

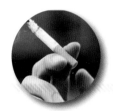

Smokers -- we all know that a smoker's lungs build up tar, and this tar leads to faster aging of the lungs.

Fast Food -- it's probably fair to say at this point that over-consumption of greasy fast food leads to clogged arteries, heart attacks, and strokes.

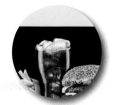

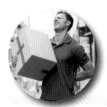

Over-exertion -- we've seen lots of cases of sudden cardiac death, either from chest trauma, overexertion, or unknown cause. In many cases, there is a link to overexertion, or one specific moment of pushing so hard that the heart fails.

Power lines & cancer -- there is strong evidence suggesting that the electromagnetic waves created by power lines leads to a change in body cells, which has an increased risk of associated cancers.

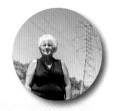

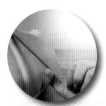

Sun exposure -- many people believe in using high-SPF sunblock; others believe that sunblock leads to cancer. Either way, there appears to be a balance -- that is unique to you, based upon your skin tone, exposure over time, and frequency of burn -- between time in the sun to boost immunity and avoiding too much sun to avoid cancer.

Oxygen -- the air we breathe has oxygen, which nourishes our bodies with every breath we take. In certain cases, environmental air can be toxic, or sub-toxic, creating massive stress on the body. The air you breathe is one very important epigenetic factor to consider, which means the location you live in predisposes you towards expressing your best or worst genes.

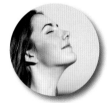

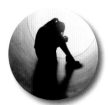

Depression & disease -- there is a strong link between 'feeling' and 'health' that is well-understood across medical practitioners. Patients who believe in themselves and have a positive attitude out-perform patients who do not believe in themselves and/or have a negative attitude, time and time again. It's clear that how you feel, on the inside, affects how you perform on the outside. time in the sun to boost immunity and avoiding too much sun to avoid cancer.

When we think of life and death circumstances, it becomes clear that our choices affect our health. However, it's the small choices that affect us in a 'small' way, throughout each and every day. For example, if you live in a city with a lot of smog, you're kind of like the smoker, except less at a time, and it's more gradual. Or if you're a professional athlete, then you're stressing your body in a life or death way on a regular basis, often asking it to perform at its maximum capacity. Either way, the choices we make affect our health, because they affect our genes on a minute-to-minute basis.

And in order to care for your body, its organs, and your health, you must first understand your body, and which systems are under greatest stress or demand. One great way to begin is by understanding body morphology, or how your body's shape and size biologically determines which bodily systems are highest functioning and most stressed.

BODY MORPHOLOGY:

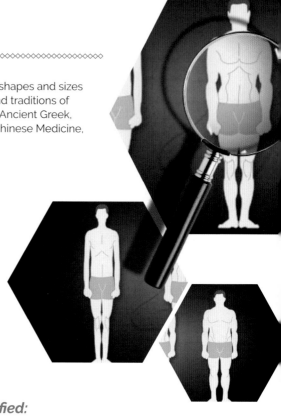

Body morphology -- or the study of body shapes and sizes -- dates back to many ancient, cultures and traditions of our past, including the Ancient Egyptians, Ancient Greek, Traditional Chinese Medicine, 5 Element Chinese Medicine, Ayurvedic Practice/traditions.

And, most indigenous cultures around the world still live this way naturally, as they have people in their villages who do more of the manual labor, strategize for food for the village, nurture children as they grow, or plan ceremonies; there are but a few examples of how applying body morphology might look in practice.

For most indigenous cultures, life path is chosen based upon biology first, rather than any other factor. It makes sense.

3 body types have been identified:

ECTOMORPH

-- long, thin bones

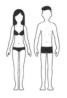

Ectomorphs are natural-born leaders, energetic beings, and purpose-driven individuals. They are often mistaken for being impersonal, although each statement made is done thoughtfully, in a calculated way. Due to busy minds and undying desire to conquer the world, ectomorphs may seem standoffish or the life of the party, depending upon what's most important to them at the time.

From a dietary standpoint, some ectomorphs do better than others with large portions of meat. In general, meat should be extremely well-cooked -- like stew meat -- and antioxidant intake should be high to balance oxidative stress to the nervous system. Fruit smoothies and veggie juices are advised. The taller and thinner the ectomorph, the hotter the environment should be, and the more time alone will be needed. The smaller-framed ectomorph will have more ability to adapt, albeit climate, activity level, diet, or relationships.

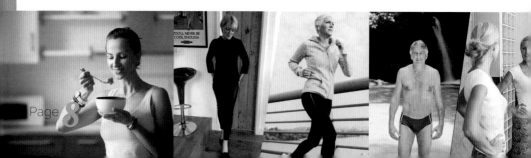

MESOMORPH

-- medium build

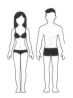

Mesomorphs are biologically lean, strong, and agile. They benefit from being active, living in warm and dry climates, and releasing energy through their upper bodies relatively early and often throughout each day. They are naturally great meat eaters and do well with 5-6 meals per day.

Mesomorphs benefit from a blend of a high antioxidant diet with a diet rich in animal-based proteins and vegetables. For this reason, salads can be a great accompaniment to any meal, and choosing the highest quality meats will make a major difference in health, due to frequency of consumption.

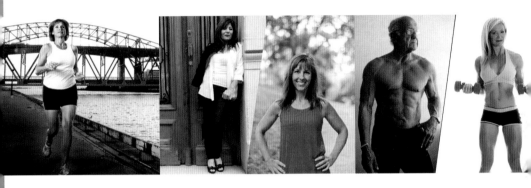

ENDOMORPH

-- thicker bones
(short or long)

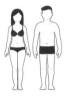

Endomorphs are bigger-boned people who tend to emphasize family, have big hearts, and are excellent with energy conservation through stored calories. Generally speaking, endomorphs function best at their own speeds, waking up later in the day, and while eating 2-3 meals per day.

Sugar is the enemy for endomorphs. Because energy is stored so easily, synthetic sugars, in particular, are like automatically-binding molecules of nastiness that attach to hips, thighs, upper arms, love handles, and the lower belly, resulting in rapid weight gain.

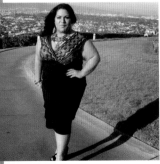
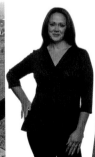
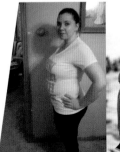
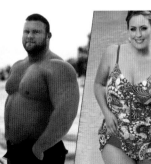

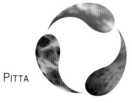

VATA

PITTA   KAPHA

Within each body type, there are sub-classifications according to each area of science that discusses them. For example, Ayurvedic medicine discusses the following body types:

paired with the element of 'air' -- is mobile, and specializes in movement + communication. Vata is creative and flexible, by nature.

☐ When unhealthy, this dosha experiences fear, anxiety, isolation, loneliness, and exhaustion.

    ○ This dosha is best paired with the Mesomorph first, and Ectomorph second.

paired with the element of 'fire' -- is transformative, and able to digest/synthesize. This dosha is known for intelligence, understanding, digestion of foods, thoughts, emotions, and experiences.

☐ When unhealthy, pitta causes fiery, reactionary emotions such as frustration, anger, jealousy, and criticism. Imbalanced pitta is often at the root of inflammatory disorders.

    ○ This dosha is best paired with the Ectomorph first, and mesomorph second.

paired with the element of 'water' -- drives community, cohesiveness, and structure. This dosha embodies love and compassion, and a healthy body maintains great immunity, as well as function in general.

☐ When unhealthy, kapha triggers emotions of attachment, greed, and possessiveness. They can also be known for stubbornness, lethargy, and resistance to change. And they will experience resistance in the mind.

    ○ This dosha is best paired with the Endomorph first, and Ectomorph second.

In ayurvedic tradition, these are referred to as 'doshas'. Each dosha corresponds with patterns and traits of an individual, likelihood of strain/disease for certain systems of the body, and natural health potential in certain areas. Interestingly, doshas also correlates with anthropometric measurements of the body, or the body's shape and size.

In Traditional Chinese Medicine (TCM), the body types are a bit different, and yet very similar:

thin, lean body types that move with grace. These people tend to be Type A, determined, and competitive, performing well under pressure.

passionate, charismatic, infectious feeling characterizes the fire type. Prominent cheek bones, well-proportioned, and extremely enthusiastic, while often talkative

When out of balance, Wood Types can be irritable, frustrated, and impatient and suffer health problems like PMS, high blood pressure, tight muscles, and headaches. Prolonged stress may result in craving alcohol or some other unhealthy vices or habits. Since the liver is the organ most closely linked with the 'wood type', anger, frustration, and intoxication are some of the most important epigenetic variables to manage.

When out of balance, Fire Types experience anxiety, insomnia, and palpitations. They're prone to overheating, and they are more prone to acne and skin rashes. And since the heart is the organ most linked to the 'Fire Type', they are prone to circulatory issues, as well.

o *The Wood Type is most closely associated with the Ectomorph.*

o *The Fire Type is most closely associated with the Mesomorph.*

biologically designed to nurture, Earth people have square faces with strong jaws and generally large features, especially their mouths. Their bodies are often thick set or curvy. They are known for their reliability and ability to gather community and create harmony.

intellectually sharp, with a high tendency for self-discipline, the Metal Types are often very successful. They like structure, and they tend to be organized and methodical. Perfectionists by nature, Metal Types are highly creative and detail-oriented. And since they are known for having super fast metabolisms, they rarely are overweight.

When out of balance, a thoughtful Earth Type can become obsessive, intrusive, and can cause worry unnecessarily. And since they wish to be needed sometimes, this can lead to codependent relationships, ultimately leading to further depletion. And since the organs most closely associated with the Earth Type are the digestive organs, they are susceptible to IBS, straining, loose stools, fatigue, and food allergies.

When out of balance, the Metal Types can allow grief and past hurt to damage relationships and result in further introversion. Since Metal Types tend to keep to themselves more than others to begin with, this can result in quite a bit of introversion. In some cases, Metal Types will replace intimacy with material things.

o *The Earth Type is most closely associated with the Endomorph.*

o *The Metal Type is most closely associated with the Ectomorph.*

Water

often with round faces and, and soft rounded bodies, Water types have large soft eyes, and they are often regarded as wise beyond their years. A water type might enjoy anonymity, and might often prefer quietness, or calmness.

When out of balance, water types may experience sore joints, or low back pain. Water Types may also be fearful, timid, and indecisive.

○ *The Water Type is most closely compared to some mix of an ectomorph and mesomorph.*

And once again, each body type corresponds with anthropometric measurements, meaning you can learn to measure and spot someone who is each body type.

Fascinating, right?

Yet, today, we pay very little attention to this in health and medicine. Somehow, with all of our advances, body morphology fell off the wayside. And yet it makes sense that if you have a super long digestive tract that it will take longer to digest food and foods like dense meats might ferment. It makes sense that you might want to eat animal-based proteins if your body naturally produces a lot of muscle, is built to sprint and be agile, and has a high level of stomach acid production. It makes sense that if you have a very sensitive gut -- meaning your nervous system tends to be on go-mode all the time, and you have a lot on your mind -- that you might want to eat well-cooked vegetables and small servings of well-cooked meats if you choose food that is more dense.

And this is all based upon how you are naturally built. Learning to understand which types of foods best nourish your body is a fun and exciting adventure into *you!* The first step is to take a deep breath. The second step is to abandon everything you 'know' to be true. The third step is to let your body tell you what's true from here on out. (and no one else)

I find the process of self-discovery to be awesome!

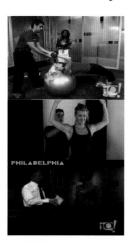

And I couldn't be more excited to share it with you.

You see, a few years ago I was teaching health at the international level, selling hundreds of thousands of copies of our top workout and diet programs, and traveling around the world healing bestselling authors, entrepreneurs, influencers, celebrities, athletes, etc. I thought I understood health, and then my intestine perforated. I became septic, meaning my body had an infection and was fighting itself; the end result: I underwent multiple organ failure.

To say the least, I was shocked to find out that what I thought to be 'the' perfect diet was awful for my body type. I was even more shocked to learn that the way my mind processes information is intense and not meant to be paired with meal time. Yet, it all made sense. I was meant to eat a variety of animal-based proteins in much smaller servings than I was eating, I was meant to eat a much larger variety of vegetables and in larger portions, and the hunch I had that fresh juice is outstanding for me turned out to be right.

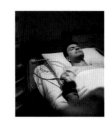

I learned all of this through developing my intuition and how it is able to guide me with food choices. I was introduced to this way of thinking by a past mentor of mine, who works with an Italian doctor named Dr. Alberto Garoli. Dr. Garoli's research integrates eastern and western medicine, ancient medical wisdoms and traditions, and modern medical advances to yield a completely personalized approach to patient care.

Dr. Garoli's research is fascinating, and it's a modern-day example of how science is catching wind of traditions from our past.

Another gentleman, Reg Lenney, spent 40 years developing his approach to health coaching, which is now completely personalized. Much like the ayurvedic, Chinese, and Dr. Garoli-ytes, Reg discovered the same basic factors that affect your health. Reg now speaks on international platforms, is the healer and health coach for pretty much every major celebrity in Hollywood, and he recently authored the book 'Be You', which details his approach to personalized health.

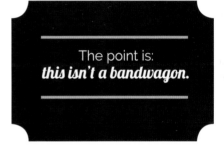

The point is: *this isn't a bandwagon.*

And you should jump on anyway. In many ways, 'real' personalized health is like the discovery of penicillin, the calorie, or the internet. Once you understand how to care for your body, in specific, life will never be the same again.

Optimal health is the beginning of life. And the easiest way to get started on your path to optimal health is to begin learning about how your body is unique and responds differently to foods than other people, even within your family.

It's a great idea to create a reset period, so to speak, so we can help ensure you're able to absorb nutrients, once you begin eating for your body. Otherwise, you could eat the perfect diet, and all the gook that built up in your gut over the years will stop you from absorbing nutrients and getting the energy you intended out of your food.

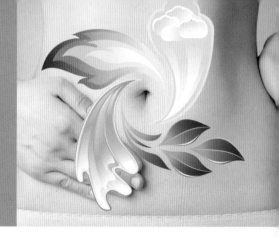

Digestive reset is why we begin with a detox. Digestive health is why there's a transition phase. And it's our view that life *begins* with optimal health, which is why there's a lifestyle section

Please enjoy My Body Cookbook. It was written for you, and with you in mind. If you have any feedback, questions, or comments, please don't hesitate to contact us:

support@createmyworkout.com

Also, if you're looking for even more personalized food recommendations, Chef Mark is the #1 resource we can share with you. Here's his contact information, and he's agreed to give discounted pricing for anyone referred by My Body Cookbook. (We do not receive any compensation for this referral.)

Chef Mark was kind enough to review, add thoughts, suggestions, and edits for every recipe in My Body Cookbook, and we are super grateful for his invaluable input. Considering the fact that he's cooked for people like Mick Jagger, the Queen, and more, I'd say we're pretty lucky to have his help.

And in spite of his success, Chef Mark keeps it real. He makes sure almost anyone can have access to personalized food coaching by offering some of the lowest rates I've seen in the industry. Please keep in mind that Mark actually spends time with each person he coaches, so this isn't some sort of lame 'fake coaching' situation where you can't get a hold of him. His prices are reasonable, and he takes the time to work with you on a personal basis. It's a sweet deal.

To get in touch with Mark, please see below:

Mark South

Email: masouth2015@hotmail.com
Skype ID: live: masouth2015
Facebook: Mark South ph360 Nutrition.

WHICH BODY TYPE ARE YOU?

Instructions:

Please choose which body type looks most like you below. You'll see there are male and female images, and each body type has examples of people who are in shape, out of shape, and obese. The reason we show you all of these examples is to also give you a visual of what your body may look like when you are super fit. Often times, we base our self-judgments upon celebrities and fitness models, who look nothing like us and have completely different bodies. Let's instead epitomize what the best version of each of us might look like.

ECTOMORPH

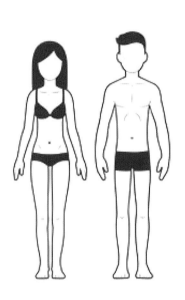

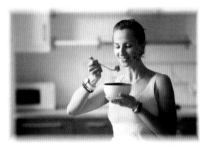

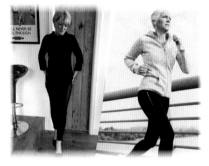

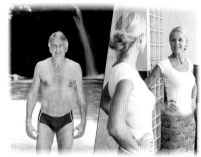

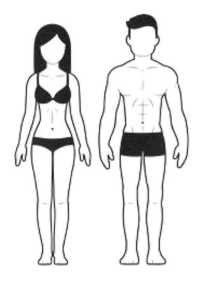

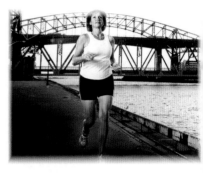

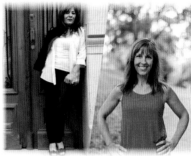

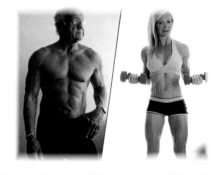

ENDOMORPH

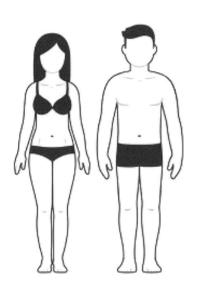
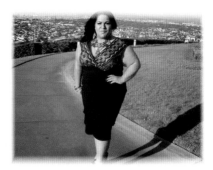
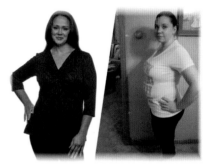
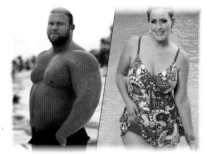

Do you know your body type?

If you're not sure, we'd love to help. In fact, we've developed
a 2 minute questionnaire that you can take by going to:
https://createmyworkout.com/personalized-health-plan.php.

NEXT STEPS ONCE YOU KNOW YOUR BODY TYPE:

1 Go to the detox section for your specific body type. (see table below for page #'s)

2 Review the recipes for your body type and go grocery shopping.

3 Plan out your meals for your detox phase, and be willing to adjust along the way.

4 Once you finish your detox phase, go to the Transition Phase for your body type.

5 After the transition phase, choose from the Lifestyle Phase recipes.

6 Learn what your body loves, or its superfoods, and bias what you eat towards these foods

Quick Reference Guide For Body Types & Recipes By Phase:

	Detox Recipes:	Transition Recipes	Lifestyle Recipes
Endomorphs:	page 20	page 46	page 124
Mesomorphs:	page 55	page 79	page 124
Ectomorphs:	page 89	page 115	page 124

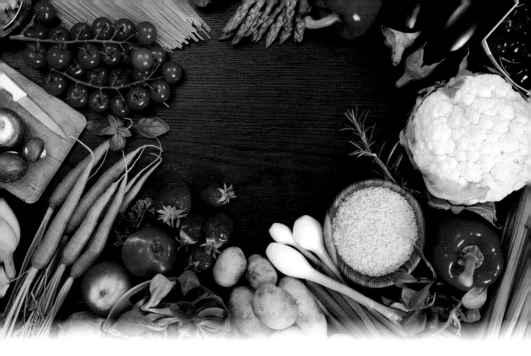

Endomorph Detox Recipes

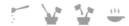

The main reasons to detox for an endomorph are to reduce circulatory stress and digestive strain. These are the two systems under greatest demand for endomorphs.

Some endomorphs tend to have longer digestive tracts, because they are taller than others. If this is the case for you, you'll want to consider a 2 week detox, rather than a 1 week detox for this phase. You see, food actually gets stuck in the digestive tract and ferments, especially dense food like animal-based protein. And this changes the way you absorb nutrients, the quality of your energy throughout the day, and your ability to heal throughout the night.

If you are a bit shorter and bigger boned (average or shorter), then one week will be plenty for your detox. Once again, your body will feel immense relief from temporarily removing animal-based protein from your diet and increasing your consumption of vegetables. You'll notice at first that you might feel famished, and then your metabolism will adjust. It typically takes 3-5 days, and once you pass this threshold, it's never the same again.

During this phase, choose freely from the recipes below. You will be eating no animal protein and minimal fats and oils, for the duration of up to a two week detox.

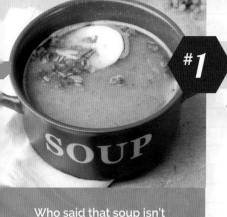

Savory Green Morning Soup

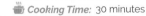

Preparation Time: 15 minutes   *Cooking Time:* 30 minutes

What's in it

Who said that soup isn't for breakfast? Enjoy this power-packed broth as a natural morning energizer. Cayenne pepper is a digestive stimulant that increases the flow of enzyme production as well as gastric juices, helping the body metabolize food and toxins. Celery is a blood cleanser and also supports healthy nervous system functioning.

2 medium yellow or green zucchini, ends cut and sliced into rounds

½ cup green string beans, ends trimmed

1 celery rib, chopped into small pieces

2 bunches curly parsley, tough stems removed

4 cups filtered water or vegetable stock

pinch of cayenne pepper

garnish with snipped chives

How to make it

Place all ingredients in a large stock pot and bring to a boil. Add cayenne pepper.

Skim the top, reduce heat and simmer for 15 minutes or until vegetables are tender.

Use a handheld blender to puree the soup, or place in batches in a tabletop blender.

Serve warm.

Dr Kareem Samhouri

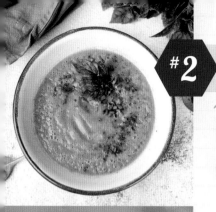

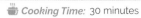

Fresh Garden Delight Soup

Preparation Time: 15 minutes   *Cooking Time:* 30 minutes

Broccoli lovers will enjoy this bold and savory mix of cleansing vegetables with just enough zip to make it a delicious dish. Broccoli is also a great source of both vitamins K and C as well as folic acid. Vitamin C protects the body from free radical damage.

What's in it

1/2 cup fresh broccoli florets

1/2 cup of celery, finely diced

½ cup leek, finely sliced

1 cup fresh spinach

1 carrot, peeled and finely chopped

3 cups organic vegetable broth

½ tsp red pepper flakes

½ lemon (juice)

garnish of snipped chives

How to make it

1. Heat 2 cups of vegetable stock in a large stock pot.
2. Add leek, carrot, celery, and broccoli. Cook over low heat for five minutes, stirring often.
3. Add the remaining vegetable broth and red pepper flakes. Bring soup to a boil and then cover and let simmer until vegetables are tender. Don't let them get mushy.
4. Add spinach.
5. Use a handheld blender or transfer to a tabletop blender. Add lemon juice to taste and process until creamy. Garnish with chives.

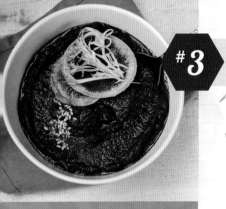

Beetsalicious Soup

Preparation Time: 15 minutes   *Cooking Time:* 45 minutes

What's in it

- 3 medium beets
- 2 medium carrots, peeled and diced
- 1 medium white onion, diced finely
- 3 garlic cloves, crushed
- 1 small leek, diced finely
- 3 cups organic vegetable broth, warmed
- ¼ tsp turmeric

How to make it

1. Fill a stock pot halfway with water. Add beets and bring to a boil. Simmer for 30 minutes or until tender.
2. Drain the beets and place them in a bowl to cool.
3. Warm 2 cups of vegetable stock in a cast iron pan, add garlic, leek, onions, and carrot. Cook for 7 minutes over low heat. Remove vegetables and put in a bowl.
4. Peel the cooled beets and cut into cubes.
5. Place the beets and vegetables into a blender along with the vegetable broth, turmeric, Process until creamy.
6. Serve warm.

Beets are loaded with vitamin C, fiber and essential minerals like potassium. Beets are known for their ability to cleanse the blood, detox the liver, and optimize the lymphatic system. This soup is so tasty, you will want to enjoy it even after the detox phase is over.

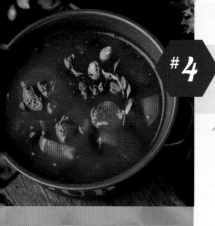

4 Cabbage and Tomato Soup
(Tailored for Endomorph)

Preparation Time: 12 minutes   *Cooking Time:* 35 minutes

What's in it

> 1 medium white onion, chopped
> 3 garlic cloves, crushed
> 1 celery rib, chopped
> 2 large carrots, sliced
> 1 15 oz can, diced tomatoes
> 6 cups organic vegetable broth
> ½ head white napa cabbage, chopped
> ¼ tsp cayenne pepper
> ¼ cup fresh basil leaves

How to make it

1. Warm 2 cups of vegetable stock in a stock pot over medium heat.
2. Add garlic, onions, celery, and carrots and simmer for five minutes or until tender.
3. Season vegetables with cayenne pepper.
4. Add the diced tomatoes and mix well.
5. Add the vegetable broth and bring to a boil.
6. Stir in the chopped cabbage and simmer for about 20 minutes until cabbage is soft.
7. Add the fresh basil to taste.
8. Serve warm.

Cabbage is one of the most potent detoxifying foods you can eat. The diuretic properties of this cruciferous veggie not only remove excess liquid from the body but also remove toxins. Cabbage also contains sulphur which helps the liver break down and release toxins.

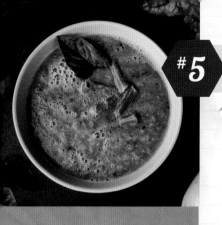

Green Beans and Basil Delight

Preparation Time: 12 minutes   *Cooking Time:* 30 minutes

What's in it

1 medium sliced leek

2 garlic cloves, crushed

1 cups fresh or frozen diced green beans

1 cup spinach

6 cups filtered water or organic vegetable stock

1 cup fresh basil leaves

1 tsp cayenne pepper

How to make it

1. Simmer 2 cups of vegetable stock and add sliced leeks, garlic and sliced cayenne until tender.
2. Add the green beans and cook for 2 minutes.
3. Add remaining water or stock and bring to a boil. Return to simmer for additional 10 minutes.
4. Allow soup to cool and pour mixture into blender.
5. Add basil leaves and spinach and blend again.
6. (Optional) For smoother consistency pass through a strainer.
7. Heat the mixture and serve.

Beans are high in fiber, and antioxidants that reduce inflammation and encourage detoxification. Basil is one herb that you can never get too much of. It has powerful antioxidant properties and helps keep the body alkaline. This soup is light but also still incredibly satisfying.

Dr Kareem Samhouri

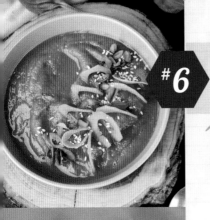

Ginger and Turmeric Carrot Soup
(Tailored for Endomorph)

Preparation Time: 15 minutes   **Cooking Time:** 30 minutes

What's in it

The therapeutic value of this delicious soup exceeds detoxification. Ginger has been shown to reduce inflammation and protect against cancer. Turmeric boosts brain health, balances blood sugar, reduces stress and relieves pain. Cayenne helps boost circulation, garlic fights bacteria and cinnamon boosts metabolism.

- 1 large white onion, diced
- 2 garlic cloves, minced
- 1-inch piece ginger, peeled and grated
- 1-inch piece turmeric, peeled and grated
- ½ tsp cinnamon
- ¼ tsp cayenne pepper
- 1 ½ pounds carrots, chopped
- 5 cups water or organic vegetable stock
- fresh chives to garnish

How to make it

1. Heat 2 cups of vegetable stock in a large stock pot, add onions and cook until slightly soft and transparent.
2. Add garlic, ginger, turmeric, cinnamon and cayenne pepper. Simmer the mixture for one minute then add the carrots and remaining liquid stock.
3. Bring mixture to a boil, reduce heat and cover. Simmer for an additional 15 minutes.
4. Soup maybe blended with hand blender until smooth or left as is,
5. Garnish with chives and serve warm.

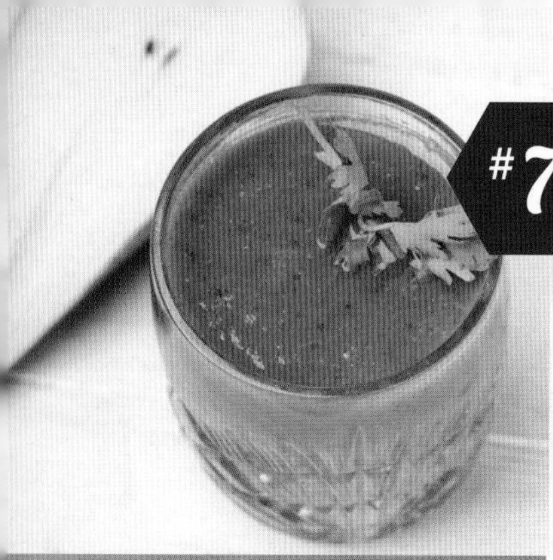

Cilantro Crush Cocktail

Preparation Time: 10 minutes   *Cooking Time:* 3 minutes

What's in it

1 bunch cilantro

2 1-inch pieces ginger

2 celery ribs

2oz or 50ml aloe vera juice pure (unsweetened)

1 pear quartered

2 whole mandarins peeled

How to make it

1. Put all ingredients through the juicer,
2. Place the cilantro, ginger, pear and mandarins in first followed by the celery to assist moving everything through juicer.
3. Add aloe vera juice to fresh juice.
4. Serve over ice.

Cilantro is loaded with healing properties that promote healthy skin and hair while reducing the risk of heart disease and diabetes. This green herb is also known for its ability to draw heavy metals from the body.

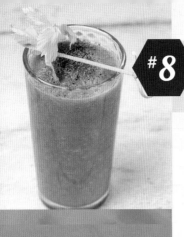

#8 Free Radical Busting Juice
(Tailored for Endomorph)

Preparation Time: 10 minutes   *Cooking Time:* 3minutes

What's in it

4 vine-ripened medium tomatoes

1 celery rib, plus leaves

½ inch knob root ginger

1 large pear

1 cup diced papaya

2 cups baby spinach

grated nutmeg

How to make it

1. Put tomatoes, celery, ginger and pear through the juicer.
2. Add the papaya and spinach to a blender and top with the fresh juice, blend until smooth.
3. Serve with a sprinkling of grated nutmeg.

This is the perfect juice to start your day or use as an energy booster before working out. Ginger is loaded with therapeutic benefits, including its ability to balance blood sugar, reduce inflammation, and support healthy digestion. Green apples are high in fiber which supports cleansing and are packed with vitamins and minerals that protect the body from free radical damage.

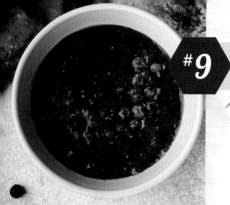

Cold Garden Greens and Blueberry Soup

✎ *Preparation Time:* 10 minutes   ☕ *Cooking Time:* 3 minutes

What's in it

1 cup baby spinach

1 cup shredded kale leaves

½ cup frozen blueberries

½ cup artichoke hearts

½ inch knob root ginger

1 cup mandarin juice

sprinkle of cinnamon

How to make it

1. Put all ingredients in blender and blend until smooth.
2. Garnish with cinnamon,

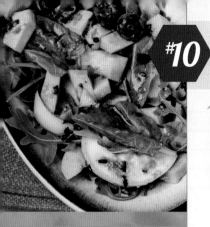

#10 Sweet Potato and Cabbage Detox Medley (AM only)

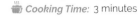

Preparation Time: 20 minutes   *Cooking Time:* 3 minutes

What's in it

> 2 large sweet potatoes, boiled lightly and cubed
>
> 2 cups baby spinach
>
> 1 cup white Napa cabbage, sliced thinly
>
> 1 cup arugula lettuce
>
> 2 eschalots sliced

Dressing

> ⅓ cup apple cider vinegar
>
> 1 tbsp honey
>
> 1 tbsp ginger, minced
>
> 1 tbsp snipped chives
>
> ½ cup frozen or fresh blueberries

How to make it

1. Combine all the lettuce leaves.
2. Blend all dressing ingredients until smooth.
3. Add sweet potatoes last.
4. Mix remaining ingredients and pour over salad.
5. Toss and enjoy.

This salad is light enough to be refreshing, yet filling enough for a meal. The combination of flavors makes it hard to believe that it is so healthy. Cabbage is known as one of the world's healthiest foods and contains over twenty different flavonoids and 15 phenols, all with immense antioxidant power. Apple cider vinegar helps regulate blood sugar and promotes healthy gut bacteria. Honey is also a famous healing food, as it is an antioxidant powerhouse and natural source of energy.

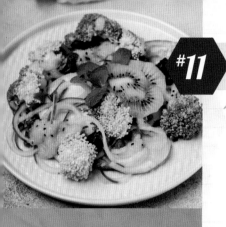

#11 Green Salad

Preparation Time: 15 minutes   *Cooking Time:* 10 minutes

Even if green is not your favorite color, you are going to love the taste of this delicious and highly nutritious salad. This salad contains vitamin-rich broccoli which contain Vitamins A and E and a host of other antioxidant powerhouses.

What's in it

¼ head green or white cabbage

¼ head broccolini

¼ cup celery, chopped

2 large cucumbers

1 lemon, juiced

1 diced eschalot

1 tsp apple cider vinegar

2 whole peeled kiwi fruits

4 half cut fresh figs

½ cup artichoke hearts

coconut water

How to make it

1. Mix the eschalot, vinegar, lemon juice and kiwi flesh in a processor and blend to smooth to make the dressing. Add a little coconut water if needed to desired consistency.
2. Make cucumber noodles with spiralizer.
3. Chop up remaining vegetables and toss them with the dressing.

Cooking Tip: To get the most juice from a lemon, roll it first, and cut it lengthwise.

Tip: For a satisfying and balanced salad for evening hours, remove all fruit and add additional greens such as asparagus and crisp green beans.

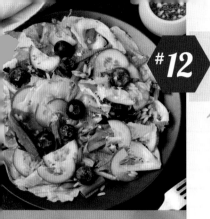

#12 Blueberry Salad
(Tailored for Endomorph)

Preparation Time: 15 minutes *Cooking Time:* 5 minutes

What's in it

For the dressing

1 tbsp lemon juice
pinch of red pepper flakes
1 tbsp rice wine vinegar
1 tsp honey
¼ tsp basil or chives
1 clove garlic, crushed

For the salad

1 cup romaine lettuce, chopped
1 cup baby spinach
1 large cucumber, chopped
½ cup fresh blueberries
½ cup shredded carrots
1 white or red onion, sliced
½ cup cooked green beans, sliced

How to make it

1. Combine all of the dressing ingredients in a shaker bottle with a lid. Shake until well blended.
2. Mix salad ingredients.
3. Pour dressing over salad and toss well.

Research has shown that eating antioxidant-rich blueberries slows the progression of liver disease as effectively as some conventional treatments. Red pepper flakes help boost immunity, aid in digestion, and control blood pressure.

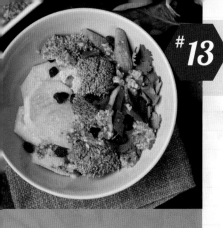

Rainbow Refreshing Mix
(Tailored for Endomorph)

🖊 *Preparation Time:* 15 minutes　　🍲 *Cooking Time:* 5 minutes

What's in it

This colorful blend will help reduce inflammation, promote healing, and cleanse your body. This salad contains cilantro (a good source of dietary fiber) as well as Vitamins A, C, E, and K along with calcium, iron, magnesium, and potassium.

For the dressing

1 tbsp apple cider vinegar
1 cup sliced cucumber
½ cup fresh cilantro
½ tbsp fresh ginger
½ tbsp raw honey
optional - coconut water if requiring a little thinning.

For the salad

1 head cooked broccoli chopped
2 cups of baby spinach
2 cups of baby carrots sliced
½ red onion sliced
⅓ cup fresh cilantro
½ cup artichoke hearts
½ cup raisins
⅛ cup sushi pink ginger
2 tsp snipped chives for garnish

How to make it

1. Add dressing ingredients to a food processor and blend to smooth.
2. Add chopped vegetables to a large bowl and mix.
3. Fold in artichoke hearts, raisins, and sushi ginger.
4. Combine ingredients for the dressing in a blender and blend until combined.
5. Pour dressing on salad and toss.
6. Garnish with chives.

Note: If you are not going to eat all of the salad at one time, keep the dressing separate from the salad.

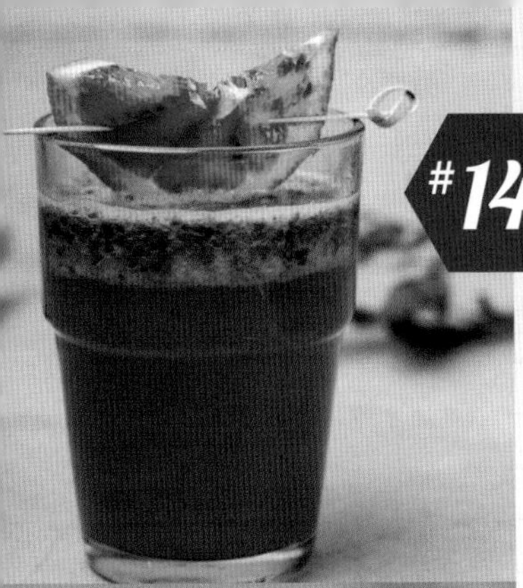

#14 Taste of the Earth Grounding Juice

Preparation Time: 8 minutes   *Cooking Time:* 3 minutes

What's in it

3 carrots

3 mandarins

2 celery ribs, with leaves

1 large green apple, quartered

a handful of organic parsley

2 fresh mint leaves

sprinkle of cinnamon

This bold juice is loaded with phytochemicals, antioxidants, and vitamins that help the kidneys flush out toxins and reduce blood pressure. Drinking this juice simply makes you feel calmer and more grounded.

How to make it

1. Mix the mandarins, carrots, celery, apple, and parsley in a juicer.
2. Grind the mint leaves with the back of a spoon and add to the juice.
3. Garnish with cinnamon sprinkle.

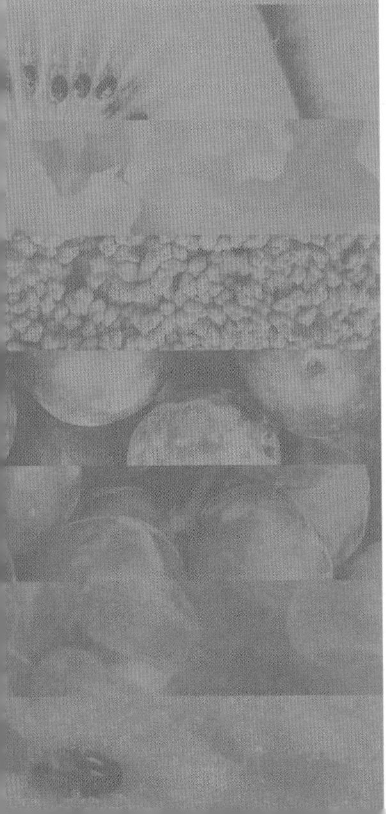

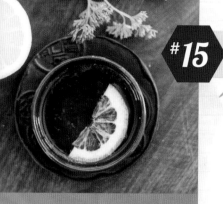

Hot Ginger Tonic

Preparation Time: 5 minutes   **Cooking Time:** 3 minutes

Ginger boosts immunity, protects against cancer, and soothes the digestive tract.

What's in it

- 50 ml or 2 oz aloe vera juice (unsweetened)
- 2 tbsp freshly grated ginger root
- 2 cups hot filtered water
- 1 tbsp raw honey

How to make it

1. Mix the juice, ginger and water together with a spoon. Add the honey until it dissolves.
2. Allow to infused for 2-3 minutes.

Dr Kareem Samhouri

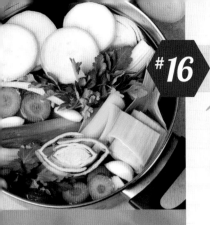

#16 Basic Clear Detox Broth

Preparation Time: 10 minutes   *Cooking Time:* 110 minutes

What's in it

1 gallon filtered water

2 large onion, chopped

3 leeks, chopped roughly

6 garlic cloves, sliced in halves

3 parsnips, chopped

4 carrot

1 bunch parsley

½ head green cabbage, chopped

1 3-inch piece of ginger root, chopped

6 celery ribs, chopped

1 tbsp ground turmeric

How to make it

1. Wash all of the vegetables. No need to peel.
2. Fill a stock pot with water and add the vegetables. Bring to a simmer, cover with a lid, and simmer for a minimum of 90 minutes.
3. Strain the liquid through a mesh strainer and discard the vegetables.
4. Store in mason jars for up to 1 week or freeze.

You can add all sorts of fun vegetables to this basic detox broth. Parsnips are a root veggie that contain large amounts of dietary fiber, potassium, magnesium, zinc, and vitamins B,C, E. Onions are rich in sulphur, which helps the body release toxins from the liver. Keep this cleansing broth on hand at all times when you need a quick pick-me-up.

#17 Berry and Spinach Special

Preparation Time: 10 minutes   *Cooking Time:* 5 minutes

Not only is this salad full of health boosting vitamins and minerals, but it is also colorful and tastes amazing. Blueberries are known for their antioxidants that have a major impact on reducing whole-body inflammation. Spinach is high in niacin and zinc as well as protein, fiber, vitamins A, C, E, K, thiamin, vitamin B6 and folate, calcium, iron, magnesium, phosphorus, potassium, copper, and manganese.

What's in it

For the dressing

2 ½ tbsp apple cider vinegar

1 tbsp honey

10 mint leaves

⅓ cup blueberries

For the salad

6 oz baby spinach

8 oz blueberries

4 oz arugula leaves

½ cup of artichoke hearts

⅓ cup sliced red onion

½ cup sliced celery

1 cup cooked diced pumpkin

How to make it

Dressing

Mix the vinegar, honey, blueberries and mint together in a food processor.
Blend until smooth.

Salad

Toss the berries and spinach together.
Add the remaining ingredients.
Drizzle with dressing and serve.

Dr Kareem Samhouri

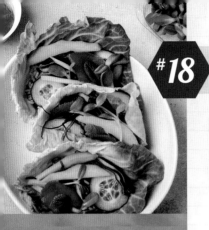

#18 Lettuce Wraps

Preparation Time: 10 minutes   *Cooking Time:* 3 minutes

What's in it

> 6 large romaine or chard leaves
> ½ cup celery, sliced thin
> 1 mango sliced
> 1 cup sprouts
> ½ cucumber, sliced thin
> 4 sliced red radishes
> pink sushi ginger to garnish
> mint leaves to garnish

These delicious wraps are easy to make and pair nicely with a bowl of veggie detox broth. Sprouts help with blood purification and boost immunity. Mangos contain tartaric acid, malic acid, and some citric acid that helps maintain the alkali reserve of the body.

How to make it

1. Lay out the lettuce leaves.
2. Divide ingredients between leaves.
3. Evenly sprinkle with vinegar, sushi ginger and mint leaves.
4. Wrap and enjoy.

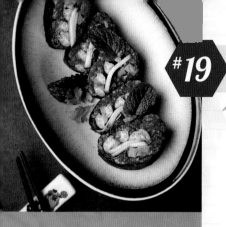

#19 Spring Nori Wraps

Preparation Time: 10 minutes　　*Cooking Time:* 5 minutes

What's in it

For the wraps

1 package of nori wraps sheets
3 cups sprouts
1 cup celery, sliced in fine strips
1 cup English cucumber, cut into matchsticks
½ buch mint, stems removed
1 bunch cilantro, stems removed
½ bunch Thai basil
½ cup of grated carrots

For the dipping sauce

1 tbsp hoisin sauce
2 tsp liquid aminos
1 tsp garlic, minced
1 tsp Sriracha sauce
2 tbsp warm water

How to make it

Sauce

Blend all ingredients together in a small bowl until desired thickness. Add more water if necessary.

Wraps

Soak each wrapper in warm water until it becomes pliable. About 45 seconds.
Lay out damp wrapper and create a base layer with sprouts.
Add carrots, celery and cucumbers. Stay about ⅓ away from edge of wrapper.
Top with some mint, basil and cilantro.
Fold over sides and bottom for a nice tight roll.
Dip in sauce and enjoy!

These satisfying little wraps contain carrots which help the liver detox, mint for optimal digestion, cucumbers for hydration, and sprouts for protein that will keep you full and satisfied. Make a batch ahead of time and enjoy them all week.

 Dr Kareem Samhouri

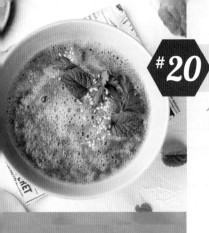

#20   *Easy Asparagus Soup*

Preparation Time: 8 minutes   *Cooking Time:* 40 minutes

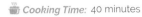

What's in it

1 small onion, chopped

1 large bunch asparagus spears, tough ends cut off and chopped

4 cups of vegetable stock

2 cup water

½ cup fresh mint leaves

½ cup fresh dill

½ cup fresh flat leaf parsley

1 head boston lettuce sliced

How to make it

Warm 2 cups vegetable stock to a large saucepan over medium heat. add onion until soft and translucent.

Add the asparagus spears. Cook on low/medium for about 2 minutes.

Add the remaining vegetable stock and bring to a boil and simmer for 15 minutes.

Add the lettuce leaves. Simmering for an additional minute.

Add fresh herbs dill, parsley and mint.

Optional - Blend the soup in a blender until smooth or serve as is.

Asparagus is a natural diuretic and can help the body remove excess salt and fluid. In addition, it helps flush toxins from the kidneys and prevent kidney stones. The mint leaves in this soup aid in digestion and support healthy detoxification.

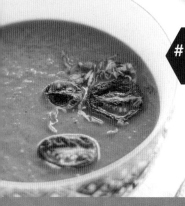

#21   Tomato Popper Soup

Preparation Time: 8 minutes   *Cooking Time:* 120 minutes

What's in it

1 pint grape tomatoes

1 tbsp ginger, minced

½ medium vidalia onion, chopped

2 tbsp garlic, minced

2 12 oz cans fire roasted diced tomatoes

1 qt organic vegetable stock

handful fresh basil

cayenne pepper to taste

2 tsp apple cider vinegar

How to make it

Warm oven to 300 degrees.

Place tomatoes on a baking pan and roast for 35 minutes. Turn off oven and allow them to sit for an additional 15 minutes. Remove any darkened skin.

Cook onions and ginger in a medium pan for a few minutes in ½ of vegetable stock.

Add the roasted tomatoes and garlic. Press down the tomatoes with the back of a spoon.

Add canned tomatoes and remaining vegetable stock. Bring to a simmer and cook for 20 minutes.

Add basil, cayenne pepper and vinegar.

Blend well with an immersion blender.

Garnish with basil sprigs.

Tomatoes are rich in lycopene which has been shown to protect against breast, skin, and lung cancer. This satisfying soup also contains ginger and garlic, two powerful detoxifiers.

Dr Kareem Samhouri

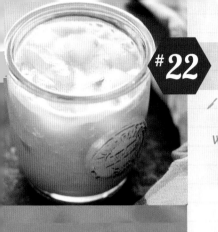

#22 Carrot and Sweet Orange Juice

Preparation Time: 3 minutes   *Cooking Time:* 3 minutes

What's in it

3 large carrots

2 tangerine or mandarins

1 blood orange

2 inch pieces of ginger

How to make it

Push all ingredients through a juicer, one at a time. Enjoy over ice.

Raw carrots contain indigestible fiber that helps the body naturally detox.

Hot and Sour Cleansing Soup

Preparation Time: 10 minutes   *Cooking Time:* 30 minutes

This inflammation-busting Asian soup has amazing flavor that will have you coming back for more. Mushrooms contain selenium, a mineral not found in most fruits and vegetables. Selenium supports liver enzyme function, helps detoxify some compounds that cause cancer, and helps prevent inflammation.

What's in it

- 1 oz dried mixed mushrooms
- 6 cups filtered water or vegetable stock
- ¼ cup apple cider vinegar
- 2 tbsp liquid aminos
- 1 tbsp ginger, minced
- 1 cup collard greens, chopped
- 1 cup sliced bok choy
- 6 scallions, trimmed and sliced thinly
- 2 cloves garlic
- ¼ tsp white pepper
- 1 jalapeno peppers, sliced

How to make it

Cover dried mushrooms with 2 cups of boiling water. Let them sit for 20 minutes. Remove the mushrooms from the water and slice them. Set the water aside.
Combine 4 cups of water and 2 cups of mushroom broth along with the sliced mushrooms, bok choy and greens in a soup pot. Bring to a boil over medium heat. Add the vinegar, aminos, garlic and ginger. Allow soup to simmer uncovered for 10 minutes.
Add the scallions and white pepper and cook for a few more minutes.
Garnish with jalapeno peppers.

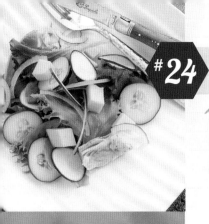

#24 Reset Salad

Preparation Time: 8 minutes   *Cooking Time:* 3 minutes

This is a super quick and easy salad that will help your body shift into detox mode.

What's in it

For the dressing

¼ cup fresh mint leaves

1 cup diced mango

1 lemon, juiced

½ tsp black pepper

For the salad

8 cups mixed greens

½ red onion, diced

4 radishes, sliced thinly

1 cup artichoke hearts

1 cup sliced cucumber

How to make it

Place greens in large serving bowl, add red onion, radishes, artichokes and cucumber.
Blend the dressing ingredients until smooth and drizzle over the leaves.
Season with pepper to taste.
Enjoy immediately.

#25 Simply Cleansing Broth

Preparation Time: 5 minutes   *Cooking Time:* 10 minutes

What's in it

    3 cups of organic vegetable broth
    ½ cup artichoke hearts
    ½ tsp freshly snipped chives

How to make it

    Warm the broth.
    Finely shredded cooked artichoke hearts.
    Snip chives.
    Place the artichokes and chives in a serving bowl and
    pour over the clear broth, serve.

On-the-go tip: Broth is ideal for the whole period of a detox, have on hand a thermos flask to enable you to warm and transport your broth with you, keeping it available at all times.

Carry your artichokes and chives separate and add to the warm broth prior to consumption.

Dr Kareem Samhouri

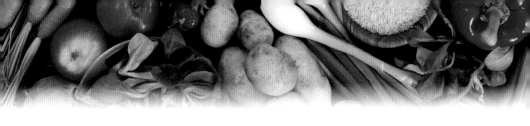

Endomorph Transition Recipes:

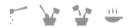

Transitioning back to a 'normal' diet that includes more protein and fat means that you're bound to increase the amount of strain on your digestive system. This also means that your heart will be working harder while your body is adapting. That's why it's a great idea to transition your diet, rather than go directly from a detox to a lifestyle plan.

During this 5 day transition phase, please choose freely from the recipes below.

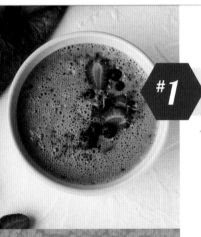

#1 Strawberry Hemp Refresher

🖊 **Preparation Time:** 5 minutes   🍲 **Cooking Time:** 3 minutes

What's in it

1 cup frozen strawberries
½ cup blueberries
1 cup coconut water
1 cup pear juice
2 tbsp hemp seeds
80ml or 3 large egg whites
grated nutmeg for topping

How to make it

Put everything in a blender and blend well.
Sprinkle with grated nutmeg.
Serve immediately.

This smoothie is a great way to start your day and will provide just the boost you need to tackle anything that comes your way. Strawberries are not only naturally sweet and delicious, but they also contain vitamin C, folate, potassium, manganese, fiber, and magnesium.

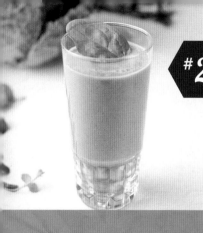

#2 Green Smoothie Deluxe
(Tailored for Endomorph)

🥄 *Preparation Time:* 5 minutes   🍲 *Cooking Time:* 3 minutes

This smoothie is creamy and very refreshing with a medley of nutrient-rich ingredients that taste amazing when blended.

What's in it

½ cup of shredded kale leaves
⅓ cup Italian, flat-leaf parsley
2 handfuls spinach
¼ avocado, medium-size
½ green apple, medium-size
½ cup diced papaya
1 tbsp flax seeds
1 cup unsweetened almond milk
¼ cup egg raw whites

How to make it

Cut any large fruits into chunks.
Place ingredients into blender and process until smooth.

Dr Kareem Samhouri

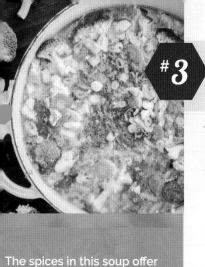

#3 Soothing Chicken Soup
(Tailored for Endomorph)

Preparation Time: 15 minutes   **Cooking Time:** 150 minutes

What's in it

2 lbs boneless chicken

8 cups chicken broth

1 cup leek, chopped

1 tsp fresh grated ginger

3 cups carrots, chopped

3 cups celery, chopped

8 cloves garlic, chopped

1 head broccoli

¼ cup snipped spring onions

½ tbsp chopped parsley

1 tsp pink himalayan salt

¼ tsp black pepper

The spices in this soup offer powerful healing properties and flavor that will have you coming back for a second bowl every time.

How to make it

Place the chicken, ginger and garlic in a large stock pot and add broth to just cover the chicken, bring to a boil. Lower the heat and simmer for 20 minutes until the chicken is entirely cooked. Remove the chicken and set aside.

Cut up vegetables while the chicken is cooking. Combine the broth with the chicken stock. Add leek, carrots and celery. Bring to a boil, reduce heat to medium and cook covered for about 10 minutes. Shred the chicken with a fork and add it to the pot, along with broccoli and parsley.

Bring the soup to a gentle boil, lower heat, and simmer covered, until all the vegetables are tender. Add salt and pepper to taste.

Garnish with the spring onions.

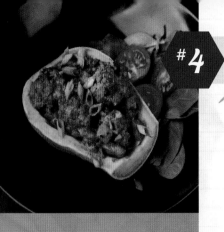

Spaghetti Squash with Bison Meatballs

Preparation Time: 10 minutes   *Cooking Time:* 60 minutes

What's in it

1-3 pounds spaghetti squash

½ cup of vegetable broth

3 tbsp of avocado oil

½ cup fresh parsley, chopped

½ tsp onion powder

1 tsp Italian seasoning

½ tsp pink himalayan salt

½ tsp black pepper

1 tbsp garlic, minced

½ tsp red pepper flakes

1 pound ground bison or veal

1 28 oz can crushed tomatoes

How to make it

Preheat oven to 375 ˚F.

Cut the squash in half, lengthwise and scoop out the seeds. Place face down in an oven safe dish and add ½ cup of vegetable broth. Cook at 375 ˚F for 30 minutes.

Warm 1 tablespoon of oil in a large skillet over medium heat. Scrape out the flesh from the squash and cook in the skillet, stir occasionally until the moisture is gone and squash begins to lightly brown.

Stir in ¼ cup parsley and remove from heat.

Combine the rest of the parsley, onion powder, salt, pepper, and ½ teaspoon Italian seasoning in a medium bowl. Add the bison/ veal and gently mix. Form meatballs from 2 tablespoons of meat.

Heat 1 tbsp oil over medium-high heat. Add the meatballs, reduce the heat and cook until brown, About 4-6 minutes. Set aside.

Add garlic to 1 tbsp of oil and cook for one minute. Add crushed tomatoes, red pepper, ½ tsp Italian seasoning and salt and pepper to taste.

Serve the meatballs over the squash and top with tomatoes.

Tip: Add a portion of steamed green leaf vegetables.

This dish has all the boldness of pasta without the carb overload. Spaghetti squash is a nutrient rich option and contains dietary fiber, vitamins C and A, along with potassium and calcium. Bison is a great source of lean protein and supports a healthy immune system while reducing inflammation. This meal is perfect for one of those days when you just need "a little more."

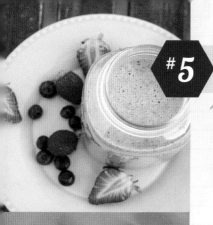

#5 Protein Packed Berry Blast

Preparation Time: 5 minutes *Cooking Time:* 3 minutes

What's in it

12 oz coconut water

1 cup spinach

2 cups frozen mixed berries

½ cup plain yogurt

1 large egg white

1 tbsp hemp seeds

1 tsp cinnamon

How to make it

Toss all ingredients in a blender and blend until smooth.
Serve immediately.

This smoothie ranks at the top of the list for its antioxidant properties.

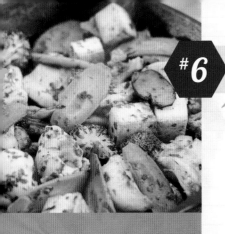

#6 Chicken and Tofu Veggie Stir Fry

Preparation Time: 12 minutes   **Cooking Time:** 10 minutes

The tofu in this recipe takes on the flavor of chicken and the vegetables offer a nice crunch. It also contains plenty of vitamins and minerals that support healing.

What's in it

3 tbsp avocado oil

1 chicken breast or thigh meat, skin removed and diced into 1-inch pieces

¼ tsp pink Himalayan sea salt

¼ tsp black pepper

¼ tsp red pepper flakes

3 oz firm tofu, cut into 1-inch cubes

1 cup broccoli florets, chopped

1 cup sliced green beans

1 cup sliced carrots

½ cup shelled edamame beans

1 tbsp raw honey

How to make it

Warm 2 tablespoons avocado oil in a pan. Add the chicken and sprinkle with salt, pepper, and red pepper flakes. Cook through and remove from heat.

Wipe the pan and add one tablespoon avocado oil. Add tofu once the oil is hot and saute by continued movement over medium heat until brown on all sides. Remove and set aside.

Add broccoli, carrots and green beans to the pan and saute until tender. Reduce the heat to medium and push all vegetables to one side of the pan.

Add the honey. Warm these together and combine the vegetables.

Stir in edamame.

Add chicken and tofu, and saute until everything is mixed.

Dr Kareem Samhouri

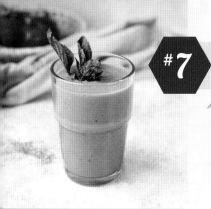

#7 Perky Pepper Smoothie

Preparation Time: 5 minutes   *Cooking Time:* 3 minutes

What's in it

1 handful of spinach
½ avocado, medium-size
2 cloves garlic
2 tomatoes
1 cups filtered water or cabbage juice
80ml or 3 large egg whites
½ cup papaya
1 green pepper, seeded
hot sauce to taste

How to make it

Toss all ingredients in a blender and blend until smooth.
Add hot sauce to taste.
Serve immediately.

Green peppers contain powerful antioxidants that boost immunity and reduce inflammation. This smoothie will wake you up in the morning and give you a healthy start to your day.

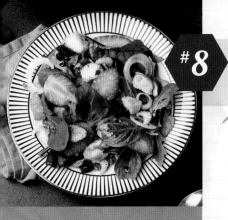

#8 Chicken and Fruit Salad - lunch only (Tailored for Endomorph)

Preparation Time: 10 minutes **Cooking Time:** 45 minutes
Includes cooking chicken within cook time

This colorful salad is full of flavor and health promoting ingredients. Tarragon triggers the stomach's natural digestive juices making it a powerful digestive aid. Plus, the balsamic vinegar adds just the right amount of zip.

What's in it

2 cups skinless chicken, roasted and sliced

2 ribs celery, chopped

1 diced eschallot

¼ cup dried cranberries

½ seeded pomegranate

30gms or ¼ cup pistachio nuts

1 tbsp fresh tarragon, chopped

1 tbsp avocado oil

1 tbsp balsamic vineger

black pepper to taste

6 cups fresh salad greens

pink himalayan salt to taste

How to make it

Mix celery, eschallots, pistachios, pomegranate and cranberries together in a large bowl along with the salad greens

Combine the tarragon, avocado oil, vinegar, and salt and pepper to create dressing.

Add the chicken to the greens and toss with the dressing.

Dr Kareem Samhouri

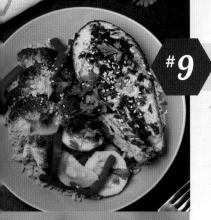

Salmon or Trout with Steamed Vegetables With Purple Rice

Preparation Time: 8 minutes   *Cooking Time:* 30 minutes

This is a very soothing and satisfying dish with plenty of flavor and nutrition. Purple rice is an excellent source of magnesium, phosphorus, selenium, thiamin, niacin, and vitamin B6.

What's in it

salmon or trout fillets 150gms or 5oz
½ cup purple rice, uncooked
1 cup napa cabbage, chopped
½ head broccoli, chopped
½ red bell pepper, chopped
2 tsp avocado oil
1 tbsp minced garlic
1 handful fresh parsley, chopped
¼ tsp cayenne pepper
2 tsp liquid aminos
sesame seeds for sprinkling

How to make it

Prepare the rice according to the package directions.
Heat oil in the wok. Add fillets face down. Cook 2 minutes and lightly turn over.
Add garlic, cayenne pepper, liquid aminos and continue to cook 2 more minutes. Add parsley.
Remove fillets from wok and set aside.
Place a little water in a wok or frying pan and bring it to a boil.
Add vegetables and cook for 2 minutes over high heat.
Place vegetables and rice on base of plate and top with fillets.
Add sesame seeds for garnish.

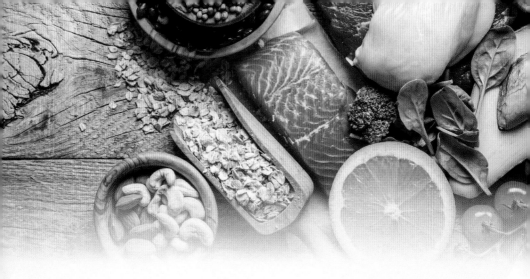

Mesomorph Detox Recipes

Mesomorphs naturally produce high levels of stomach acid, making for a natural ability and inclination to eat meat and other dense proteins. The biological design of a mesomorph allows you to move quickly, be agile, and naturally develop strength that make your friends jealous.

Mesomorphs are also natural feelers, meaning they are incredibly gifted with emotions and emotional intelligence. They can sense and detect the slightest change in mood, energy, or emotion. And with all of this in mind, it's important to have fun during a detox if you're a mesomorph, and it's important to feel great.

This means it's time to rest on eating dense proteins, eliminate meat for 3 days if you're a bit shorter (with rounder hips), and eliminate protein for 4 days if your natural body build is a V-shape and you find it particularly easy to build muscle definition when you do the work.

During this three to four day detox phase, you can choose freely from the recipes below. You will be consuming no animal protein and minimal fats and oils during this phase.

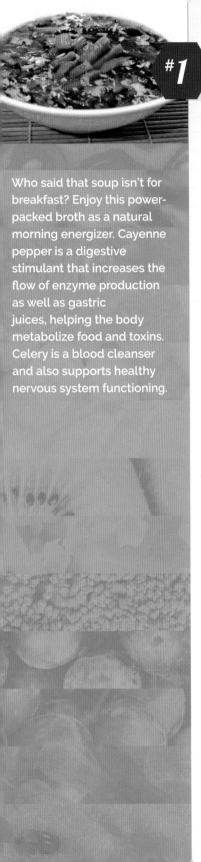

Savory Green Morning Soup

Preparation Time: 10 minutes   *Cooking Time:* 30 minutes

Who said that soup isn't for breakfast? Enjoy this power-packed broth as a natural morning energizer. Cayenne pepper is a digestive stimulant that increases the flow of enzyme production as well as gastric juices, helping the body metabolize food and toxins. Celery is a blood cleanser and also supports healthy nervous system functioning.

What's in it

- 4 medium zucchini, ends cut and sliced into rounds
- 1 lb green string beans, ends trimmed
- 2 celery ribs, chopped into small pieces
- 2 bunches curly parsley, tough stems removed
- 4 cups fresh carrot juice
- pinch of cayenne pepper

How to make it

Place all ingredients in a large stock pot and bring to a boil. Add cayenne pepper.

Skim the top, reduce heat and simmer for 15 minutes or until vegetables are tender.

Serve warm.

Optional: Use a handheld blender to puree the soup, or place in batches in blender.

Garden Delight Soup

Preparation Time: 8 minutes   *Cooking Time:* 10 minutes

Broccoli lovers will enjoy this bold and savory mix of cleansing vegetables with just enough zip to make it a delicious dish. Broccoli is also a great source of both vitamins K and C as well as folic acid. Vitamin C protects the body from free radical damage.

What's in it

- ½ cup fresh broccoli florets
- 1 rib celery, finely diced
- 1 whole leek, finely sliced
- 1 cup fresh baby spinach
- 1 carrot, peeled and finely chopped
- 2 cups organic vegetable stock
- ½ tsp red pepper flakes
- snipped chives to garnish

How to make it

Heat a shallow amount of broth in a large stock pot. Add leek, carrot, celery, and broccoli. Cook over low heat until carrot become soft.

Add the remaining vegetable broth and red pepper flakes. Bring soup to a boil and then cover and let simmer for 2 minutes. Don't let them get mushy.

Add the spinach.

Add chives to garnish and serve.

Dr Kareem Samhouri

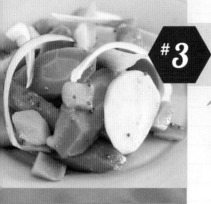

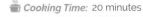

Nothing But Roots Salad
(Tailored for Mesomorph)

Preparation Time: 10 minutes   **Cooking Time:** 20 minutes

What's in it

1 red onion diced

1 butternut squash, sliced into sections

1 carrot, cut into bite-size pieces

1 parsnip, cut into bite-size pieces

1 celery rib, cut into bite-size pieces

1 teaspoon balsamic vinegar

1/2 teaspoon mustard seeds

1 tsp raw honey

1 handful parsley leaves

2 tsp lemon juice

How to make it

Cook all vegetable in shallow water just covering the vegetables, until ⅔ soft cooked.

Whisk the vinegar, lemon juice, honey and mustard seed in a large bowl to create the dressing and combine it with the vegetables. Add any additional seasonings you desire for taste.

Serve warm. Sprinkled with parsley.

Not only is this salad filling and delicious, but it is also loaded with cleansing root vegetables that scrub your digestive tract, build your immune system, and help reduce free radicals. Enjoy as a meal or an anytime snack.

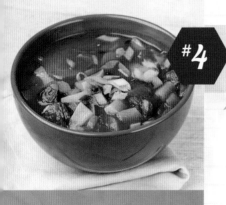

Cabbage Soup
(Tailored for Mesomorph)

Preparation Time: 12 minutes   **Cooking Time:** 40 minutes

What's in it

1 medium white onion, chopped

3 garlic cloves, crushed

3 ribs celery, chopped

3 large carrots, sliced

1 15 oz can, diced tomatoes

6 cups vegetable broth

½ head green cabbage, chopped

¼ tsp cayenne pepper

¼ cup basil leaves

Cabbage is one of the most potent detoxifying foods you can eat. The diuretic properties of this cruciferous veggie not only removes excess liquid from the body but also removes toxins. Cabbage also contains sulphur which helps the liver break down and release toxins.

How to make it

Add a shallow amount of stock in a stock pot over medium heat.

Add garlic, onions, celery, and carrots and cook for 2 minutes or until the onion is tender.

Season vegetables with basil and cayenne pepper.

Add the diced tomatoes and mix well.

Add the remaining vegetable broth and bring to a boil.

Stir in the chopped cabbage and simmer for about 20 minutes until cabbage is soft.

Add more seasonings to taste.

Serve warm.

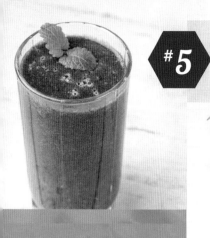

#5 Ultimate Apple and Berry Cleansing Smoothie
(Tailored for Mesomorph)

Preparation Time: 3 minutes *Cooking Time:* 3 minutes

What's in it

1 cup mixed frozen berries, like raspberries, strawberries, and blueberries

1 large apple

2 cups spinach

10ml or 1 inch knob of freshly pressed ginger juice

1 cup fresh orange juice

How to make it

Add all ingredients to a blender. Blend until smooth. Serve immediately.

Apples are a good source of vitamins A, E, K, C, and B- complex. They are also rich in polyphenols which act as antioxidants, and pectin that cleanses blood vessels of plaque. Berries are fruit superstars that are loaded with vitamins and minerals to help support the body in detoxification while boosting the immune system.

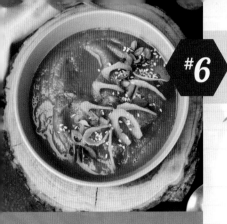

#6 Ginger, Turmeric and Carrot Soup
(Tailored for Mesomorph)

Preparation Time: 10 minutes   **Cooking Time:** 20 minutes

What's in it

1 large white onion, diced
2 garlic cloves, minced
1-inch piece ginger, peeled and grated
1-inch piece turmeric, peeled and grated
½ tsp cinnamon
¼ tsp cayenne pepper
1 ½ pounds carrots, chopped
5 cups coconut water
fresh herbs to garnish
black pepper to taste
salt to taste

How to make it

Heat 2 cups of coconut water and add the onion in a large stock pot until onion is slightly transparent.
Add garlic, ginger, turmeric, cinnamon and cayenne pepper. Simmer the mixture for 1 minute, then add the carrots and remaining coconut water.
Bring mixture to a boil, reduce heat and cover. Simmer for five minutes.
Blend with hand blender until smooth.
Add pepper and salt to taste.
Garnish with fresh herbs and serve warm.

The therapeutic value of this delicious soup exceeds detoxification. Ginger has been shown to reduce inflammation and protect against cancer. Turmeric boosts brain health, balances blood sugar, reduces stress, and relieves pain. Cayenne helps boost circulation, garlic fights bacteria, and cinnamon boosts metabolism.

Dr Kareem Samhouri

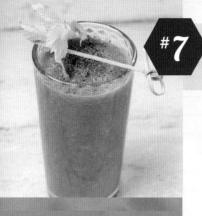

#7 Free Radical Busting Juice
(Tailored for Mesomorph)

Preparation Time: 3 minutes *Cooking Time:* 3 minutes

What's in it

3 vine-ripened tomatoes
1 celery rib, plus leaves
½ inch knob ginger
1 large green apple
ice cubes

How to make it

Put all ingredients through the juicer.
Serve over ice with celery for garnish.

This is the perfect juice to start your day or use as an energy booster before working out. Ginger is loaded with therapeutic benefits, including its ability to balance blood sugar, reduce inflammation, and support healthy digestion. Green apples are high in fiber which supports cleansing and are packed with vitamins and minerals that protect the body from free radical damage.

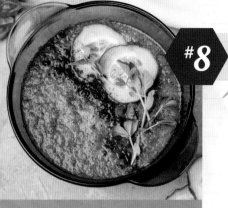

#8   *Cold Cucumber and Spinach Soup*

Preparation Time: 5 minutes   *Cooking Time:* 3 minutes

What's in it

- 1 large cucumber, peeled and deseeded
- 2 cups of baby spinach
- 1 tbsp fresh onion, minced
- 1 tbsp lemon juice
- 1 tbsp apple cider vinegar
- 1 cup coconut water
- ¼ tsp chili powder
- dash cayenne pepper
- paprika for garnish

How to make it

Put all ingredients in a blender and blend until smooth. Garnish with extra cucumber and paprika, if desired.

Tip: Soup can be warmed through if desired.

Cucumbers are rich in vitamins B, potassium, and magnesium and also contain a great deal of water which makes them a great addition to any detox diet.

Dr Kareem Samhouri

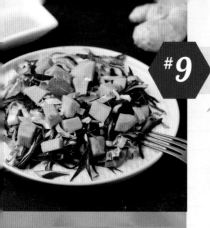

#9   Butternut Pumpkin Detox Medley

Preparation Time: 10 minutes   *Cooking Time:* 20 minutes

This salad is light enough to be refreshing, yet filling enough for a meal. The combination of flavors makes it hard to believe that it is so healthy. Cabbage is known as one of the world's healthiest foods and contains over twenty different flavonoids and 15 phenols, all with immense antioxidant power. Apple cider vinegar helps regulate blood sugar and promotes healthy gut bacteria. Honey is also a famous healing food, as it is an antioxidant powerhouse and natural source of energy.

What's in it

For the salad

2 cups diced butternut squash

3 cups kale, chopped

2 cups red cabbage, sliced thinly

For the dressing

½ cup lemon juice

1 tbsp honey

1 tbsp ginger, minced

⅓ cup apple cider vinegar

How to make it

Blanch kale and refrigerate until cool.

Cook the butternut squash, boiled lightly.

Combine red cabbage with kale.

Add sweet butternut squash last.

Combine dressing ingredients and pour over salad.

Toss and enjoy.

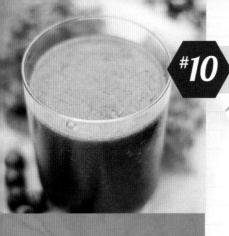

#10 Kale and Papaya Superdrink

Preparation Time: 5 minutes   *Cooking Time:* 3 minutes

What's in it

1 cup diced papaya
1 ½ cups of pear juice
1 cup frozen blueberries
1 cup kale, finely shredded
1 cup baby spinach
nutmeg sprinkled

How to make it

Add all ingredients to a blender. Blend until smooth.
Sprinkle with nutmeg.
Serve immediately.

Kale is loaded with calcium, vitamin A, vitamins C, E, B6, and K, folic acid, iron, potassium, magnesium, zinc, and sodium.

Dr Kareem Samhouri

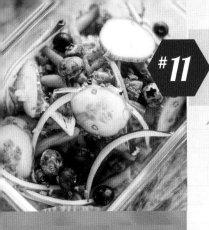

#11

Blueberry Bliss Salad
(Tailored for Mesomorph)

 Preparation Time: 10 minutes   *Cooking Time:* 20 minutes

What's in it

For the dressing

> pinch of red pepper flakes
> 1 tsp honey
> 1 tsp chopped chives
> ½ cup blueberries

For the salad

> 1 cup romaine lettuce, chopped
> 1 cup baby spinach
> 1 large cucumber, chopped
> ½ cup fresh blueberries
> ½ cup shredded carrots
> ½ red onions, sliced
> ½ cup green beans, sliced

How to make it

> Combine all of the dressing ingredients in a blender until smooth.
> Mix salad ingredients.
> Pour dressing over salad and toss well.

Research has shown that eating antioxidant-rich blueberries slows the progression of liver disease as effectively as some conventional treatments. Red pepper flakes help boost immunity, aid in digestion, and control blood pressure.

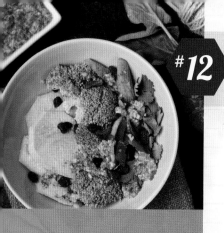

#12 Rainbow Refreshing Mix
(Tailored for Mesomorph)

Preparation Time: 10 minutes   *Cooking Time:* 5 minutes

What's in it

For the dressing

⅓ cup apple cider vinegar
½ tbsp fresh cilantro
½ tbsp fresh ginger
1 tbsp raw honey
¼ tsp black pepper

For the salad

1 head cauliflower, chopped
2 cups red cabbage, finely sliced
2 cups baby carrots, finely sliced
½ red onion, sliced
⅓ cup fresh cilantro
½ cup of diced papaya
1/4 cup raisins

How to make it

Add dressing ingredients to a food processor.
Add chopped vegetables to a large bowl and mix.
Fold in the papaya and raisins.
Pour dressing on salad and toss.

Note: If you are not going to eat all of the salad at one time, keep the dressing separate from the salad.

This colorful blend will help reduce inflammation, promote healing, and cleanse your body. This salad contains cilantro (a good source of dietary fiber) as well as Vitamins A, C, E, and K along with calcium, iron, magnesium, and potassium. Kale aids in digestion and has more iron than beef.

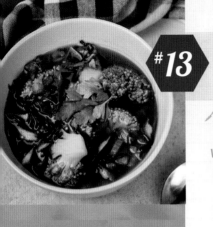

#13 Hearty Vegetable Soup
(Tailored for Mesomorph)

Preparation Time: 15 minutes   **Cooking Time:** 35 minutes

This colorful soup is not only beautiful, but is also warm, healthy, and delicious. The energizing ingredients work together to support a healthy detox. Carrots help boost immunity, aid in digestion, reduce macular degeneration, and support healthy blood pressure.

What's in it

½ red onion, diced
2 tbsp garlic, minced
3 celery ribs, diced
3 medium carrots, diced
1 small head of broccoli florets
1 cup tomatoes, chopped
1 tbsp fresh ginger, peeled and minced
1 tsp powdered turmeric
1/4 tsp cinnamon
1/8 tsp cayenne pepper
6 cups vegetable broth
2 cups kale, de-stemmed and torn into pieces
1 cup purple cabbage, chopped
salt to taste
pepper to taste

How to make it

Add ¼ cup broth to large stock pot and heat.
Once hot, add the onion and garlic and simmer for 2 minutes.
Add celery, carrots, broccoli, tomatoes, and ginger.
Cook for 3 minutes and add in ¼ cup more vegetable broth.
Stir in turmeric, cinnamon, cayenne pepper, salt and pepper.
Pour in remaining broth and bring the soup to a boil.
Let it simmer for 10 minutes or until the vegetables are soft.
Add the kale and cabbage toward the last 3 minutes.

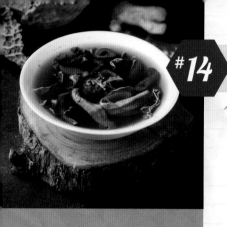

#14 Hot and Sour Cleansing Soup

Preparation Time: 10 minutes　　*Cooking Time:* 30 minutes

What's in it

- 1 oz dried mixed mushrooms
- 2 cups filtered water
- 4 cups vegetable stock
- ¼ cup apple cider vinegar
- 2 tbsp liquid aminos
- 1 tbsp ginger, minced
- ½ cup collard greens, chopped
- 6 scallions, trimmed and sliced thinly
- 2 cloves garlic
- ¼ tsp white pepper
- 1 jalapeno, sliced
- ½ tsp of salt

How to make it

Cover dried mushrooms with 2 cups of boiling water. Let them sit for 20 minutes. Remove the mushrooms from the water and slice them. Set the water aside.

Combine 4 cups of vegetable stock and 2 cups of mushroom broth along with the sliced mushrooms and greens in a soup pot. Bring to a boil over medium heat. Add the vinegar, aminos, salt, garlic and ginger, allow soup to simmer uncovered for 10 minutes.

Add the scallions and white pepper and cook for a few more minutes.

This inflammation-busting Asian soup has amazing flavor that will have you coming back for more. Mushrooms contain selenium, a mineral not found in most fruits and vegetables. Selenium supports liver enzyme function, helps detoxify some compounds that cause cancer, and helps prevent inflammation.

Dr Kareem Samhouri

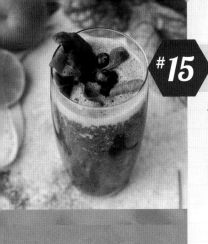

#15 Fruit Surprise

Preparation Time: 5 minutes   *Cooking Time:* 3 minutes

The refreshing nature of this delicious drink is complimented by its potent immune supporting and cleansing power.

What's in it

1 cup freshly squeezed orange juice
1/2 cup carrot juice
½ cup blueberries
½ cup papaya
½-inch ginger sliced
1 cup baby spinach
1 cup arugula leaves

How to make it

Add all ingredients to a blender. Blend until smooth. Serve immediately.

Turnip Treat

Preparation Time: 5 minutes *Cooking Time:* 3 minutes

What's in it

- ½ turnip
- 3 carrots
- 1 green apple
- ¼ fennel bulb
- 1 tsp lime juice
- 2 mandarins
- sprinkle of ground cinnamon

How to make it

Chop all ingredients and put through your juicer. Serve over ice and sprinkle with cinnamon. Drink immediately.

Even if you are not a big fan of turnips, you will love this tasty vitamin C rich drink. It is so easy to make and contains ingredients that will help boost your eyesight, prevent kidney stones, lower cholesterol and even help keep cancer at bay.

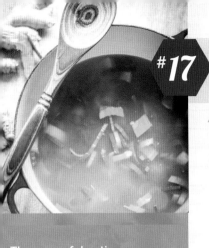

#17

Golden Goodness Broth
(Tailored for Mesomorph)

Preparation Time: 8 minutes   *Cooking Time:* 15 minutes

The powerful anti-inflammatory nature of turmeric and ginger combined with the antioxidant properties of onion give this simple to make broth the power to support your body during detox.

What's in it

1 leek, diced
2 tbsp fresh ginger, grated
3 tsp fresh turmeric, grated
1 tsp ground cumin
1 tsp ground coriander
4 cups water
4 cups vegetable stock
¼ tsp cayenne pepper
3 tsp apple cider vinegar

How to make it

Add 2 cups of vegetable stock to a medium pan and heat to simmering point, add leek and cook to slightly soft,
Add ginger and lower the heat to a light simmer.
Add spices and cook for one more minute while stirring.
Add the remaining vegetable stock and water. Bring broth to a simmer and add the vinegar.
Season to taste.

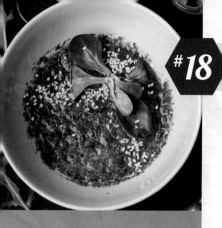

Super Green Broth

Preparation Time: 5 minutes   **Cooking Time:** 5 minutes

What's in it

- 1 cup vegetable broth
- 1 cup arugula leaves
- 2 tbsp tarragon, chopped
- 2 tbsp chervil, chopped
- 2 tbsp chives, chopped
- 1 cup shredded artichoke hearts

How to make it

Warm the vegetable broth until hot.

Add all ingredients into a blender, except artichokes.

Pour the broth in and blend until frothy.

Add artichokes.

Serve and enjoy.

Don't let the green color fool you, this is a delicious and cleansing soup. Arugula is loaded with powerful antioxidants. The vitamins and nutrients in this broth will boost your immune system functioning, increase your metabolism, improve mineral absorption and improve your energy.

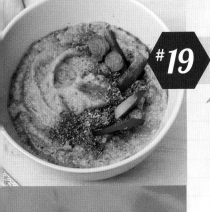

#19 Cauliflower and Broccoli soup

Preparation Time: 10 minutes **Cooking Time:** 35 minutes

This soup contains B vitamins riboflavin, niacin and thiamine. It is bursting with a robust flavor that will make you forget you are on a detox. The dietary fiber in this soup will keep your digestive system functioning smoothly and the vitamin C is important for immune health.

What's in it

1 medium onion, chopped

2 garlic cloves, grated

½ tsp salt

½ tsp pepper

1 cauliflower head, cut into florets

2 broccoli heads cut into florets, slice steams

4 cups vegetable broth

1 tbsp dried mint

How to make it

Place the onion, garlic, salt and pepper in 2 cups of vegetable stock over medium heat and simmer for 3 minutes.

Add cauliflower, broccoli and remaining vegetable stock.

Bring back to boil and reduce to simmer with lid on for about 15 minutes.

Remove from the heat and use a hand blender to blend well.

Add the dried mint and blend until smooth.

Add seasoning to taste.

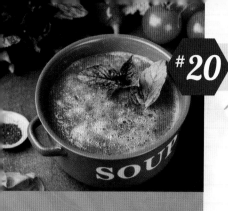

#20 Tomato Popper Soup

Preparation Time: 8 minutes   *Cooking Time:* 120 minutes

Tomatoes are rich in lycopene which has been shown to protect against breast, skin, and lung cancer. This satisfying soup also contains ginger and garlic, two powerful detoxifiers.

What's in it

- 1 pint grape tomatoes
- 1 tbsp ginger, minced
- ½ medium vidalia onion, chopped
- 2 tbsp garlic, minced
- 2 12 oz cans fire roasted diced tomatoes
- 1 qt or 4 cups vegetable stock
- handful fresh basil
- 2 tsp apple cider vinegar
- cayenne pepper to taste

How to make it

Warm oven to 300 degrees.

Place tomatoes on a baking pan and roast for 35 minutes. Turn off oven and allow them to sit for an additional 15 minutes. Remove any darkened skin.

Cook onions and ginger in a medium pan for a few minutes in 2 cups of vegetable stock.

Add the roasted tomatoes and garlic. Press down the tomatoes with the back of a spoon.

Add canned tomatoes and remaining vegetable stock. Bring to a simmer and cook for 20 minutes.

Add basil, cayenne pepper and vinegar.

Blend well with an immersion blender.

Garnish with basil sprigs.

 Dr Kareem Samhouri

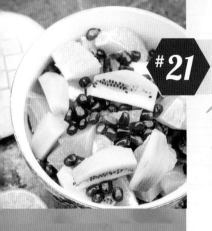

#21 Power Fruit Medley - Ideal for a Morning Starter

Preparation Time: 10 minutes *Cooking Time:* 3 minutes

What's in it

> 1 cup black grapes, cut in half and deseeded
> 1 small pineapple, peeled and cut into 1-inch chunks
> 4 small clementines, peeled and segmented
> 2 apples, cored and cut into 1-inch pieces
> 1 orange, peeled and cut into 1-inch chunks
> 2 kiwi fruits, peeled and cut into 1-inch chunks
> 1 mango, peeled and cut into 1-inch chunks
> seeds of 1 pomegranate
> juice of 1 orange

How to make it

> Add all the fruit apart from the pomegranate to a large bowl.
> Pour the juice over the fruit and top with the pomegranate seeds.

Grapes are high in minerals, organic acids and grapeseed oil that can have a positive impact on health. Pineapple contains bromelain, a powerful digestive enzyme and anti-inflammatory. Pomegranates also have three times the amount of antioxidants than red wine and green tea.

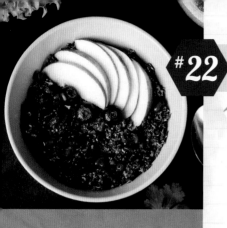

#22 Mother Earth Delight

Preparation Time: 10 minutes   *Cooking Time:* 3 minutes

Don't let the sweet and crunchy taste of this earth salad fool you. It is loaded with vitamins and minerals to support healthy digestion and cleansing. Make a big batch and munch on it all week.

What's in it

2 heads broccoli

1 cups kale, chopped

1 cups red cabbage, chopped

1 cup baby spinach

2 cups baby carrots

1/2 of a red onion

1/3 cup fresh cilantro, de-stemmed and chopped

1/2 cup pomegranate seeds

Garnish

1 apple, diced

2/3 cup fresh blueberries

balsamic vinegar, to taste

How to make it

Shred or slice broccoli, kale, cabbage, carrots, onion and cilantro.

Add to a large bowl and mix in baby spinach and pomegranate seeds.

Drizzle with balsamic vinegar. Add fresh fruits garnish.

Dr Kareem Samhouri

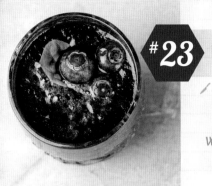

#23 Blueberry Blend

Preparation Time: 10 minutes   *Cooking Time:* 3 minutes

This detox blend will give you a great burst of energy in the morning or is perfect for an afternoon pick-me-up.

What's in it

1 cup blueberries
1 whole fig (when available)
1 cup baby spinach
2 cups carrot and orange juice
10 ml or 1 inch knob of pressed ginger
½ cup artichoke hearts
ground cinnamon to garnish

How to make it

Toss all ingredients into a blender and blend well.
Sprinkle with cinnamon.
Enjoy immediately.

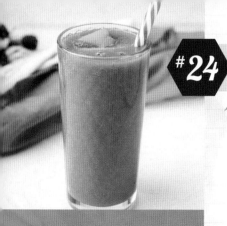

#24 Sweet Papaya Smoothie

/ **Preparation Time:** 8 minutes　　**Cooking Time:** 3 minutes

What's in it

1 cup papaya
1 cup coconut water
1 cup carrot juice
1 cup baby spinach
1 cup of shredded kale

How to make it

Place all ingredients into a blender and blend until smooth.
Serve immediately.

Papaya contains a powerful digestive enzyme known as papain that helps support natural detoxification. This tropical fruit also reduces inflammation and purifies the blood.

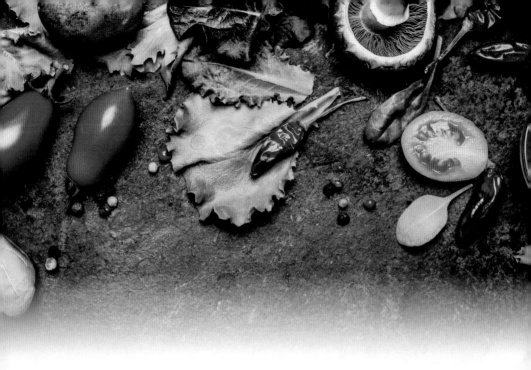

Mesomorph Transition Recipes

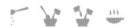

It doesn't take very long for your system to begin producing normal to high levels of stomach acid if you're a mesomorph. In fact, it seems to only takes about one day, although we find that allowing 3 days to transition your diet is much more comfortable and enjoyable, from a digestive habits standpoint.

During this 72 hour transition, be sure to at least drink 64 ounces of water and enjoy herbal tea.

Exercise lightly and get plenty of sleep.

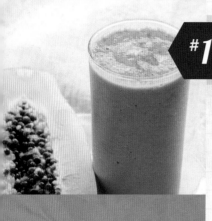

Green Smoothie Deluxe
(Tailored for Mesomorph)

#1

Preparation Time: 5 minutes   *Cooking Time:* 3 minutes

What's in it

⅓ cup Italian, flat-leaf parsley

2 handfuls baby spinach

¼ avocado

½ cup of diced papaya

1 tbsp hemp seeds

1 cup orange juice

10ml or 1 inch knob of pressed ginger

80ml or 3 large egg whites

How to make it

Place all ingredients into a food processor and blend until smooth.

Add additional liquid to adjust to prefered consistency and serve.

This smoothie is creamy and very refreshing with a medley of nutrient-rich ingredients that taste amazing when blended.

Physique Cookbook | Dr Kareem Samhouri

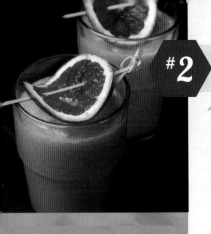

#2 Orange Turmeric Reboot

Preparation Time: 5 minutes   *Cooking Time:* 3 minutes

What's in it

3 large carrots

3 oranges

2 cups baby spinach

½ inch turmeric root

½ inch ginger root

How to make it

Peel orange and cut all ingredients to fit through your juicer.

Juice and serve over ice if preferred.

This warming juice will promote healthy liver function and ease your digestive system.

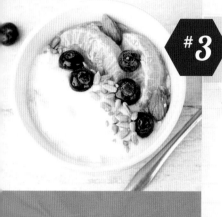

Tropical Fruit, Nut and Yogurt Treat

Preparation Time: 5 minutes   *Cooking Time:* 3 minutes

What's in it

- 1/2 cup goat, sheep or coconut yogurt
- 1/4 cup fresh blueberries
- 2 tsps linseed, almond and sunflower mix (LSA)
- 1 mandarin segmented
- 1 ½ tbsp raw honey
- nutmeg to garnish

How to make it

Place yogurt in the base of a serving bowl and top with remaining ingredients.
Top with nutmeg.

Tartaric acid, malic acid, and citric acid found in blueberries help preserve alkali reserves.

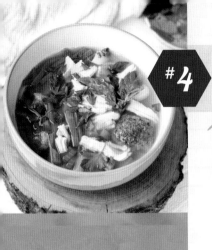

Soothing Chicken Soup
(Tailored for Mesomorph)

Preparation Time: 15 minutes   *Cooking Time:* 50 minutes

What's in it

- 2 lbs boneless chicken
- 8 cups chicken broth
- 1 cup leek, chopped
- 3 cups carrots, chopped
- 3 cups celery, chopped
- 1 cup broccoli florets
- ¼ cup snipped spring onions
- ½ tbsp parsley, chopped
- 1 tsp pink Himalayan salt
- ¼ tsp black pepper

The spices in this soup offer powerful healing properties and flavor that will have you coming back for a second bowl every time.

How to make it

Place the chicken in a large stock pot and add water to just cover the chicken, bring to a boil. Lower the heat and simmer for 20 minutes until the chicken is entirely cooked. Remove the chicken and set aside.

Cut up vegetables while the chicken is cooking. Combine the broth with the chicken stock. Add leek, carrots and celery. Bring to a boil, reduce heat to medium, and cook covered for about 10 minutes.

Shred the chicken with a fork and add it to the pot, along with broccoli and parsley.

Bring the soup to a gentle boil, lower heat, and simmer covered, until all the vegetables are tender. Add salt and pepper to taste.

Garnish with the spring onions.

#5 Tuna and Tomato Wrap

Preparation Time: 10 minutes   *Cooking Time:* 3 minutes

What's in it

1 can solid white tuna, drained
½ small avocado, smashed
2 tbsp hummus
6 cherry tomatoes, chopped
1 gluten-free wrap of your choice
handful of baby spinach

How to make it

Combine the drained tuna, hummus, tomatoes and avocado in a bowl.
Add the baby spinach to ⅓ of the wrap.
Top with the tuna mixture and roll.

This is a perfect and simple lunch that will leave you satisfied and energized. Tuna contains omega-3 fatty acids which help to keep blood vessels healthy, reduce cholesterol in arteries, and lower blood pressure.

Dr Kareem Samhouri

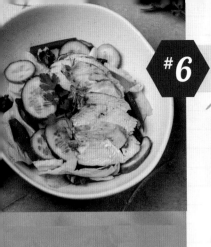

#6 Organic Chicken Salad Bowl

Preparation Time: 10 minutes   *Cooking Time:* 15 minutes

This beautiful chicken salad bowl combines powerful antioxidants with turmeric, a potent anti inflammatory spice.

What's in it

For the dressing

1 garlic clove, minced

2 tbsp apple cider vinegar

½ tsp sea salt

¼ tsp black pepper

1 tsp extra virgin olive oil

½ tbsp raw honey

For the salad

1 boneless, organic skinless chicken breasts

½ tbsp olive oil

1 tsp ground turmeric

1 garlic clove, minced

sea salt and pepper to taste

¼ cup pecans, chopped

½ large head Romaine lettuce, chopped

½ small red onion, sliced

½ English cucumber, sliced

½ red bell pepper, sliced

How to make it

Combine the oil, turmeric, garlic, sea salt and pepper in a medium bowl. Toss well.

Preheat a skillet over medium heat and add the chicken. Cook through, cool and cut into small pieces.

Whisk the dressing ingredients in a small bowl.

Add salad ingredients and chicken to the medium bowl.

When you are ready to eat the salad, pour the vinaigrette dressing over the salad and toss well.

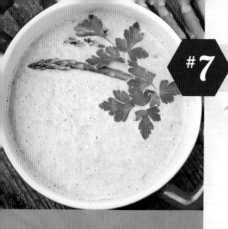

#7 Asparagus Soup

Preparation Time: 8 minutes   *Cooking Time:* 40 minutes

This warm and creamy soup has a slightly tropical taste and makes a perfect dinner alone or paired with gluten-free bread. Coconut butter is rich in lauric acid, a powerful immune system booster. It also destroys harmful bacteria, viruses, and fungus.

What's in it

2 tbsp coconut butter

1 garlic clove, minced

2 lb. asparagus, ends trimmed into 1" pieces

sea salt, to taste

ground black pepper, to taste

1 cup chicken broth

½ flax or almond milk

chopped fresh chives for garnish

chopped dill for garnish

How to make it

Melt butter in a heavy pot over medium heat. Add garlic and cook until fragrant.

Add the asparagus and season with salt and pepper. Gently cook for about 5 minutes.

Add broth and simmer uncovered about 10 minutes.

Blend the soup with an immersion blender or put into tabletop blender

Return to pot and add in the milk. Warm over low heat. Garnish and serve.

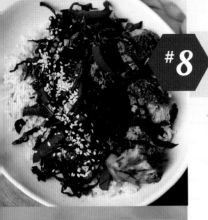

#8 Steamed Vegetables With Brown Rice

Preparation Time: 10 minutes   *Cooking Time:* 35 minutes

This is a very soothing and satisfying dish with plenty of flavor and nutrition. Brown rice is an excellent source of magnesium, phosphorus, selenium, thiamin, niacin, and vitamin B6. It also promotes the release of melatonin to aid in restful sleep. It is recommended to eat 2-3 hours prior to resting.

What's in it

½ cup brown rice, uncooked
1 cup red cabbage, chopped
½ head broccoli, chopped
½ red bell pepper, chopped
2 tsp avocado oil
1 tbsp minced garlic
1 handful fresh parsley, chopped
¼ tsp cayenne powder
2 tsp liquid aminos
sesame seeds for sprinkling

How to make it

Prepare the rice according to the package directions.
Place a little water in a wok or frying pan and bring it to a boil.
Add vegetables and cook for 2 minutes over high heat.
Drain and set aside.
Heat avocado oil in the wok and add garlic, cayenne powder, and parsley.
Add the vegetables and liquid aminos. Cook for 2 minutes.
Serve over the brown rice.
Add sesame seeds for garnish.

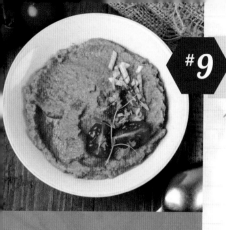

Roasted Tomato and Cauliflower Soup

/ **Preparation Time:** 10 minutes   **Cooking Time:** 30 minutes

This creamy, yet dairy-free soup is full of bold flavors. Shallots are one of the most powerful antioxidant foods and contain healing sulfur compounds. Pair with a side salad for a perfect light dinner.

What's in it

- 1 pint cherry tomatoes
- 1 head cauliflower, cut into bite sized florets
- 2 tbsp rice bran oil
- 1 whole shallot, chopped fine
- 2 cloves garlic, minced
- 6 cups vegetable broth
- 3 sprigs thyme for garnishing, chopped
- 3 whole bay leaves
- ½ tsp sea salt
- ¼ tsp black pepper

How to make it

Preheat oven to 400 F. Toss tomatoes and cauliflower in a large roasting pan with 1 ½ tbsp oil. Roast for 10 minutes or until the tomatoes blister and the cauliflower is softened.

Saute the shallot in the remaining ½ tbsp oil until fragrant. Add the garlic and cook for about a minute more. Stir frequently.

Combine the tomatoes, cauliflower, shallot, garlic, broth, thyme, bay leaves, and salt and pepper. Simmer for about 10 minutes, stir occasionally. Remove bay leaves.

Blend soup with an immersion blender or blend in parts in a table top blender

Add additional warm broth to desired consistency. Serve immediately.

Dr Kareem Samhouri

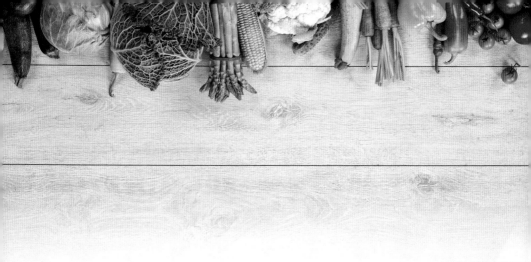

Ectomorph Detox Recipes

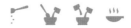

Ectomorphs are thinkers, by nature, which means they have highly programmed nervous systems. Some ectomorphs are taller and thinner than others, as a result of having the fastest metabolisms. For this reason, they can get away with a one-day detox and simply eliminating protein, while increasing well-cooked vegetables consumption for the day.

Other ectomorphs are a bit shorter, or more v-shaped and muscular. In this case, it's recommended a detox last four days, where days 1 and 3 are without protein. Elimination of proteins -- while eating a healthy diet full of natural sugars, fruits, and vegetables -- serves to take strain off the nervous system and remove toxicity. Nervous system toxicity is perhaps the #1 risk factor for ectomorphs, so making sure to do a detox quarterly is recommended.

During this one-to-four-day phase, choose freely from the below recipes, but avoid eating protein on days 1 and 3.

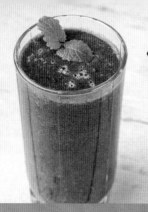

Ultimate Apple and Berry Cleansing (Tailored for Ectomorph)

Preparation Time: 5 minutes   *Cooking Time:* 3 minutes

What's in it

- 1 cup mixed frozen berries, like raspberries, blackberries, and blueberries
- 1 large apple
- 2 cups baby spinach
- 1 tbsp raw honey
- 1 cup carrot and orange juice
- 10ml or 1 inch knob presses ginger root

Apples are a good source of vitamins A, E, K, C, and B- complex. They are also rich in polyphenols which act as antioxidants, and pectin that cleanses blood vessels of plaque. Berries are fruit superstars that are loaded with vitamins and minerals to help support the body in detoxification while boosting the immune system.

How to make it

Add all ingredients to a blender. Blend until smooth. Serve immediately.

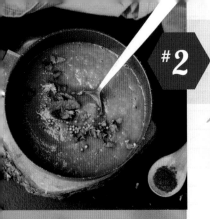

Ginger and Turmeric Carrot and Sweet Potato Soup (Tailored for Ectomorph)

#2

Preparation Time: 12 minutes *Cooking Time:* 40 minutes

The therapeutic value of this delicious soup exceeds detoxification. Ginger has been shown to reduce inflammation and protect against cancer. Turmeric boosts brain health, balances blood sugar, reduces stress and relieves pain. Cayenne helps boost circulation, garlic fights bacteria and cinnamon boosts metabolism.

What's in it

1 large leek, diced

1-inch piece ginger, peeled and grated

1-inch piece turmeric, peeled and grated

½ tsp cinnamon

¼ tsp cayenne pepper

1 ½ pounds carrots, chopped

1 pound peeled and diced sweet potato

5 cups vegetable stock

2 cloves of garlice, sliced

fresh chives to garnish

How to make it

Heat 2 cups of vegetable stock in a large stock pot add leek and cook until slightly transparent.

Add garlic, ginger, turmeric, cinnamon and cayenne pepper. Simmer for one minute,

Add the carrots, sweet potatoes and remaining stock. Bring mixture to a boil, reduce heat and cover. Simmer for twenty minutes.

Blend with hand blender until smooth.

Garnish with fresh herbs and serve warm.

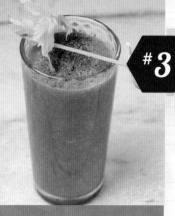

Free Radical Busting Juice
(Tailored for Ectomorph)

🖊 *Preparation Time:* 3 minutes   ☕ *Cooking Time:* 3 minutes

What's in it

3 vine-ripened tomatoes
1 celery rib, plus leaves
1 cup baby spinach
½ cup artichoke hearts
½ inch knob root ginger
1 cup carrot juice

This is the perfect juice to start your day or use as an energy booster before working out. Ginger is loaded with therapeutic benefits, including its ability to balance blood sugar, reduce inflammation, and support healthy digestion.

How to make it

Put celery, tomatoes, ginger and carrots through the juicer.
Place spinach and artichokes in a blender and top with the fresh juice, blend until smooth.

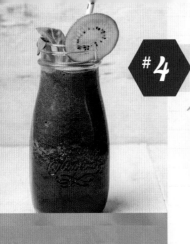

Kale and Papaya Superdrink

/ Preparation Time: 5 minutes　　*Cooking Time:* 3 minutes

Kale is loaded with calcium, vitamin A, vitamins C, E, B6, and K, folic acid, iron, potassium, magnesium, zinc, and sodium. Papaya contains a powerful digestive enzyme known as papain that helps support natural detoxification. This tropical fruit also reduces inflammation and purifies the blood.

What's in it

1 cup of diced papaya

1 cup frozen cherries

1 cup kale, chopped

1 cup arugula lettuce leaves

10ml or 1 inch knob presses ginger root

1 cup carrot juice

How to make it

Add all ingredients to a blender. Blend until smooth. Serve immediately.

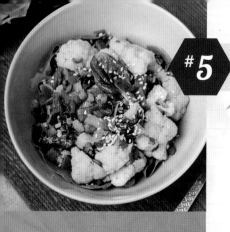

Mixed Turmeric Veggie Casserole

Preparation Time: 10 minutes   *Cooking Time:* 15 minutes

What's in it

- ½ cup carrots, peeled and chopped
- ½ cup diced fennel heart
- ½ cup sliced green beans
- 1 cup baby spinach
- 1 whole leek sliced
- 1 tsp ground turmeric
- 1 tsp ground cumin
- 1 ½ cups vegetable stock
- 1 cup butter beans
- garlic chives for garnish

How to make it

Warm stock in a braising pan, add leek, turmeric, cumin and carrots and simmer for 5 minutes,

Add the fennel and green beans and simmer for an additional 5 minutes.

Stir in the butter beans and spinach leaves and cook for one minute.

Check that carrots are tender and serve.

Top with snipped chives.

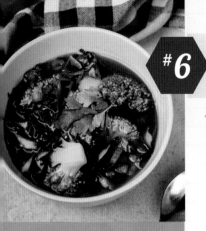

Hearty Vegetable Soup
(Tailored for Ectomorph)

Preparation Time: 15 minutes   *Cooking Time:* 40 minutes

This colorful soup is not only beautiful, but is also warm, healthy, and delicious. The energizing ingredients work together to support a healthy detox. Carrots help boost immunity, aid in digestion, reduce macular degeneration, and support healthy blood pressure.

What's in it

- 1 leek, diced
- 2 tbsp garlic, minced
- 3 celery ribs, diced
- 3 medium carrots, diced
- 1 small head of broccoli florets
- 1 cup tomatoes, chopped
- 1 tbsp fresh ginger, peeled and minced
- 1 tsp powdered turmeric
- 1/4 tsp cinnamon
- 1/8 tsp cayenne pepper
- 6 cups vegetable broth
- 2 cups kale, de-stemmed and torn into pieces
- 1 cup purple cabbage, chopped
- 1 cup diced Russet potatoes

How to make it

Add 2 cups of broth to large stock pot and heat.
Once hot, add the leek and garlic and simmer for 2 minutes.
Add the potatoes and carrots simmer 10 minutes,
Add celery, broccoli, tomatoes, and ginger. Cook for 3 minutes and add in ¼ cup more vegetable broth.
Stir in turmeric, cinnamon, cayenne pepper.
Pour in additional broth and bring the soup to a boil.
Let it simmer for 10 minutes or until the vegetables are soft.
Add the kale and cabbage toward the last 3 minutes.

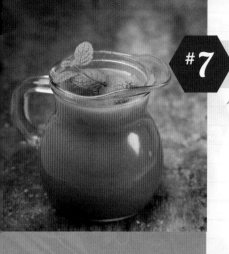

#7 Spicy Carrot Ginger Tonic

Preparation Time: 5 minutes   *Cooking Time:* 3 minutes

Ginger is the king of detox spices. Not only will this refreshing drink awaken your taste buds, but it is also a powerful anti inflammatory agent.

What's in it

- ½ inch piece ginger, minced
- 1 tsp cinnamon
- 1 tsp raw honey
- 1 handful baby spinach
- 1 cup carrot juice

How to make it

Add all ingredients to a blender. Blend until smooth. Serve immediately.

Dr Kareem Samhouri

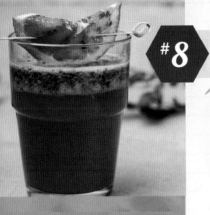

#8 AM Cleansing Juice

Preparation Time: 7 minutes   *Cooking Time:* 5 minutes

An ideal morning energy cleansing cocktail, that also provides organs to relax and release unwanted toxins.

What's in it

- 2 large carrots
- ⅛ green cabbage
- 2 peeled mandarins
- 1 peeled blood orange
- 2 celery ribs
- 30ml or 1 oz of pure aloe vera juice (unsweetened)
- 1 pear, medium
- 1 knob of fresh ginger root

How to make it

Juice all ingredients, placing the cabbage leaves, pear, mandarins, orange and ginger in first, then utilise the carrots and celery ribs to push all of the ingredients.
Stir in the aloe vera juice.
Serve immediately.

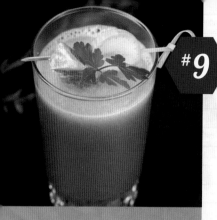

#9 PM Cleansing Juice

Preparation Time: 5 minutes   *Cooking Time:* 3 minutes

The ingredients in this juice capture the ability to influence the body to relax while providing nutrition. Cabbage provides B12 and vitamin K, while celery is a natural source of phosphorus. Carrots have many antioxidants that can help keep a body healthy. Aloe Vera contains several antioxidant properties.

What's in it

2 celery ribs
2 large carrots
1 cup cabbage
1 inch knob of fresh root ginger
½ cup cold green tea
30ml or 1 oz of aloe vera juice unsweetened

How to make it

Juice all ingredients, utilising the carrots and celery alternatively to help push through the cabbage and ginger,
Add the tea and aloe vera juice to the pressed juice, stir and serve immediately.

Dr Kareem Samhouri

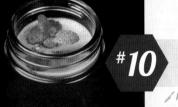

#10   Earthy Red Cleansing Juice

Preparation Time: 5 minutes   *Cooking Time:* 3 minutes

What's in it

1 green apple, cored

1 lemon, rind removed

1/2 English cucumber, cut into pieces

1 handful baby spinach

½ cup blackberries

1/2 red beet, cut into pieces

1/2-inch piece ginger root, plus more to taste, cut into pieces

How to make it

Push all ingredients through your juicer.

Enjoy immediately over ice.

This powerful cleansing drink has a sweet taste and is full of antioxidants and fiber to support a healthy detox. Apples are loaded with digestive tract cleaning fiber, while raspberries not only satisfy a sweet fix but also offer up a healthy dose of vitamin C.

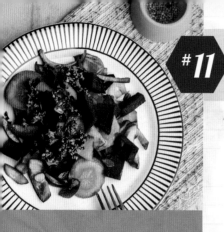

Nothing But Roots warm Salad
(Tailored for Ectomorph)

Preparation Time: 15 minutes   **Cooking Time:** 30 minutes

What's in it

- 1 red onion, sliced
- 2 whole sweet potatoes peeled and diced
- 1 butternut squash, sliced into sections
- 2 carrots, diced into 1-inch pieces
- 1 medium parsnip, peeled and diced into 1-inch pieces
- 2 celery ribs, diced into 1-inch pieces
- 1 large beet, peeled and diced into 1-inch pieces
- avocado oil for coating
- 1 teaspoon apple cider vinegar
- 1 lemon, juiced
- 1 tsp mustard powder
- 1 handful parsley leaves

How to make it

Preheat oven to 425 °F.
Coat the sweet potatoes, carrots, squash, parsnip and beet root with minimal oil
Roast until partly tender.
Add celery and onions and continue to cook until all vegetables are tender.
Whisk the vinegar, lemon juice, and mustard powder in a large bowl. Combine the dressing with vegetables.
Garnish with parsley.
Serve warm.

Not only is this salad filling and delicious, but it is also loaded with cleansing root vegetables that scrub your digestive tract, build your immune system, and help reduce free radicals. Enjoy as a meal or an anytime snack.

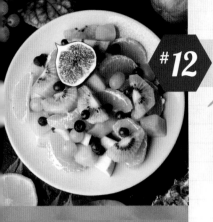

#12   Flushing Fruit Salad

Preparation Time: 12 minutes   *Cooking Time:* 3 minutes

What's in it

1 small pineapple, peeled and cut into 1-inch chunks
2 green apples, cored and cut into 1-inch pieces
4 small clementines, peeled and segmented
2 kiwi fruit, peeled and cut into 1-inch pieces
1 navel orange, peeled and cut into 1-inch chunks
1 mango, peeled and cut into 1-inch pieces
20 seedless grapes, cut in half
seeds of one pomegranate
1 orange, juiced
ground cinammon, optional topping

How to make it

Add all fruit to a large glass bowl.
Drizzle the orange juice over the fruit and mix.
Add the pomegranate seeds.
Sprinkle with cinammon if desired and gently mix.

Make a big bowl of this antioxidant fruit salad and snack on it whenever your sweet tooth starts to get the upper hand. Pineapple is a delicious tropical fruit that boosts immunity, improves blood circulation, reduces inflammation in joints, and helps improve oral and eye health. Kiwis may be small but they offer a powerful vitamin C punch, while pomegranate seeds tackle oxidative stress like a champ.

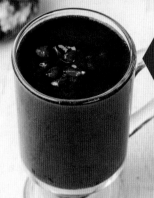

#13 Minimalist Smoothie

Preparation Time: 5 minutes   **Cooking Time:** 3 minutes

Don't let the simplicity of this smoothie fool you. Its' big taste is matched by its' whole-food goodness.

What's in it

- 1 cup mixed berries, frozen
- 1 cup baby spinach
- ½ cup diced papaya
- 1 cup arugula leaves
- 1 cup pomegranate juice, unsweetened
- 1 tsp raw honey

How to make it

Add all ingredients to a blender and blend until smooth.

Add more juice if you would like it thinner.

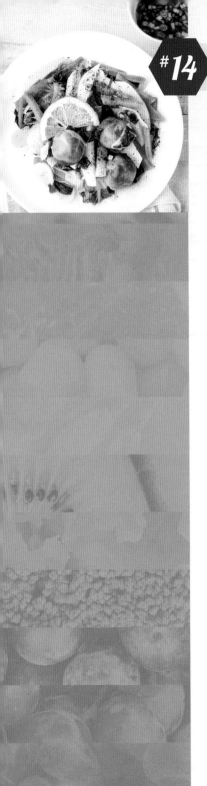

#14 Super Salad

Preparation Time: 10 minutes   *Cooking Time:* 15 minutes

What's in it

For the dressing

3 tablespoons red wine vinegar

1 1/2 tbsp honey

1 tsp snipped chives

For the salad

4 large carrots, peeled and sliced

1 cup of baby spinach

1 cup shredded kale

½ cup sprouts

1 cup diced Russet potatoes

1 leek diced

2oz of vegetable stock

How to make it

Steam carrots and potatoes until lightly tender.

In a braising dish, add stock and bring to the simmer.

Add leeks and slowly simmer for 1 minute.

Add kale and stir through then add the spinach.

Add the carrots and potatoes to the greens and stir through. Top with sprouts.

Combine dressing ingredients and drizzle over vegetables.

Serve.

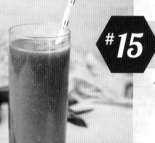

#15 Ginger and Coconut Smoothie

Preparation Time: 3 minutes   *Cooking Time:* 3 minutes

What's in it

- 1 cup of baby spinach
- 1 cup chopped romaine lettuce
- 1 cup coconut water, chilled
- 1 cup sweet blood orange juice
- 1 inch fresh ginger, peeled and chopped
- 1 bunch fresh mint

How to make it

Place all ingredients in a blender and blend until smooth.
Enjoy over ice.

This smoothie is perfect for busting the bloat. The ginger and coconut together give this drink a refreshing, tropical taste. Coconut water has been prized by islanders for hundreds of years. It is a powerful source of potassium and has even been used as a replacement for blood plasma during war stricken times.

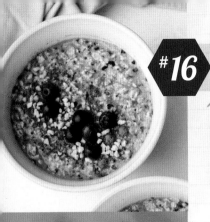

#16 Blueberry and Oats Bowl

Preparation Time: 5 minutes   *Cooking Time:* 45 minutes

An important element for ectomorph bodies during a cleanse is to still supply the body and more importantly the mind with carbohydrates, important when tasks need to be completed.

What's in it

2 cups fresh or frozen blueberries
⅔ cup coconut water
2 tbsp honey
1 banana, peeled
⅓ cup quick-cooking oatmeal
dash of cinnamon

How to make it

Blend blueberries, coconut water, honey and banana in a blender. Blend until smooth.
Divide this mixture between two bowls.
Stir in the oatmeal.
Top with cinnamon.
Put in the fridge for 30 minutes and enjoy.

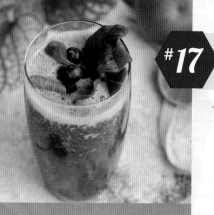

#17 Fruit Surprise

Preparation Time: 5 minutes   **Cooking Time:** 3 minutes

The refreshing nature of this delicious drink is complimented by its potent immune supporting and cleansing power.

What's in it

1 cup freshly squeezed orange juice
1/2 cup purified water
½ cup banana
½ cup strawberries
½-inch ginger peeled and sliced
1 tbsp flax oil
1 tbsp lecithin granules
1 tbsp lemon juice
1 tbsp spirulina powder
1 tbsp raw honey

How to make it

Add all ingredients to a blender. Blend until smooth. Serve immediately.

Dr Kareem Samhouri

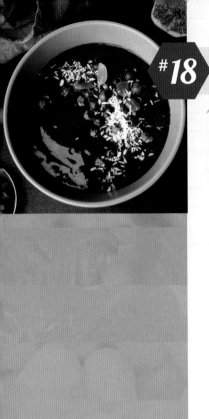

#18 Bountiful Smoothie Bowl

Preparation Time: 10 minutes *Cooking Time:* 3 minutes

What's in it

1 cup organic baby spinach

1 cup of kale

1/4 cup pitted cherries fresh or frozen

1 banana sliced, frozen

1 1/2 cups frozen organic berries

juice from 1/2 lemon

1 cup mandarin juice

pinch of turmeric optional

1 tsp raw honey

cinammon topping sprinkle

How to make it

Put all ingredients into a blender and blend until smooth. Add more liquid if needed.

Sprinkle cinammon on top.

Serve.

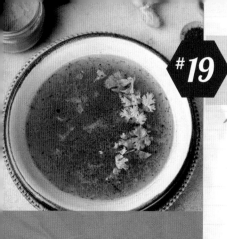

Golden Goodness Broth
(Tailored for Ectomorph)

Preparation Time: 5 minutes   **Cooking Time:** 20 minutes

What's in it

- 50ml vegetable broth
- 1 white onion, diced
- 2 tbsp fresh ginger, grated
- 3 tsp fresh turmeric, grated
- 1 tsp cumin
- 1 tsp coriander
- 1 tsp salt
- 6 cups vegetable stock
- ¼ tsp cayenne pepper
- 1 tsp lemon juice

The powerful anti-inflammatory nature of turmeric and ginger combined with the antioxidant properties of onion give this simple to make broth the power to support your body during detox.

How to make it

Saute onion in oil for about 3 minutes.

Add ginger and lower the heat. Saute the ginger with the onion until brown.

Add spices and cook for one more minute while stirring.

Add vegetable stock and bring broth to a simmer for about 10 minutes and add the lemon juice.

Season to taste.

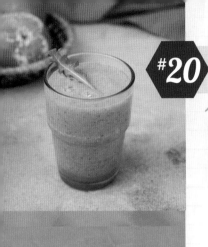

Mandarin Cleansing Mix

Preparation Time: 5 minutes *Cooking Time:* 3 minutes

Mandarin oranges are an excellent source of Vitamin C and add just the right amount of sweetness to this cleansing drink.

What's in it

3 medium green apples
1 large cucumber
1 large lemon, peeled
1 lime, including skin
3 small mandarins, peeled
1 full head romaine lettuce

How to make it

Put all ingredients through a juicer.
Serve immediately over ice.

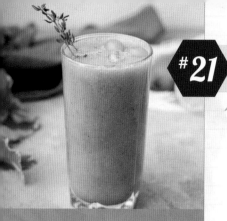

Easy Peasy Morning Juice

Preparation Time: 5 minutes   **Cooking Time:** 3 minutes

What's in it

3 ribs of celery

1/2 large cucumber, cut into quarters

1 medium green apple, cut into eighths

1 medium pear, cut into eighths

1 inch knob of fresh ginger

The quercetin content of celery along with fiber helps to clear the digestive track and supports protection from oxidative stress. This is a quick and easy solution when you're on the go.

How to make it

Put all ingredients through a juicer.
Serve immediately over ice.

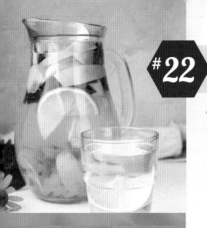

#22 Coconut Cleansing Water

Preparation Time: 5 minutes   *Cooking Time:* Overnight

One of the best ways to support healthy and natural detoxification is by consuming the proper amount of water. Coconut water, suped up with the nutrients from a variety of fruit, helps your body stay hydrated and offers a vitamin punch to support a healthy immune system. Sip on this delicious and refreshing water throughout the day or take some with you to the gym to enjoy while you workout.

What's in it

- 12 ounces of coconut water
- ½ cup of filtered water
- 1 green apple, chopped
- juice from 1 small lime
- juice from 1 small lemon
- ¼ cup of mint leaves
- 3 cups of pineapple chunks
- 1 lime, cut and peeled
- 1 lemon, cut and peeled

How to make it

Put all ingredients in a clean glass jar. Cover and place in refrigerator overnight.
Strain the water and enjoy.

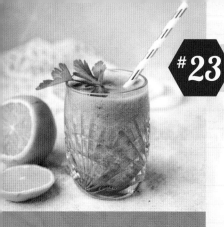

#23 Love Your Liver Smoothie

Preparation Time: 5 minutes   *Cooking Time:* 3 minutes

What's in it

> 2 oranges, peeled
> 1/2 rib celery
> 1 lemon, peeled
> 1/2 cup dandelion greens
> 1/2 cup parsley

How to make it

> Place all ingredients into a blender and blend until smooth.
> Serve immediately.

Celery may seem innocent enough however, it is loaded with powerful antioxidants and fiber that help support cleansing. Dandelion greens are rich in vitamins A, B, C and K and can help reduce inflammation and regulate blood pressure.

#24 Zesty Tomato Juice

Preparation Time: 5 minutes   *Cooking Time:* 3 minutes

What's in it

- 3 large tomatoes
- 3 celery ribs
- 2 large carrots
- 1-2 fresh chiles

How to make it

Place all ingredients into a blender and blend until smooth.
Serve immediately over ice.

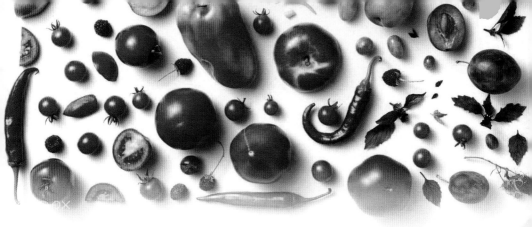

Ectomorph Transition Recipes

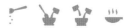

During this 72 hour transition, be sure to at drink at least 64 ounces of water and enjoy herbal or green tea. Exercise lightly and get plenty of sleep. A calm mind, as you transition back into 'normal life', may be your greatest asset. There's plenty of time for all that's to come. Right now, it's about regeneration and pause.

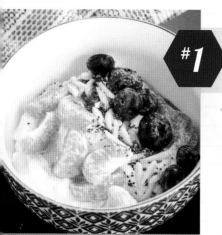

#1 Tropical Fruit, Nut and Yogurt Treat

Preparation Time: 5 minutes   *Cooking Time:* 3 minutes

What's in it

1/2 cup goat, sheep or coconut yogurt
1/4 cup fresh blueberries
2 tsps linseed, almond and sunflower mix (LSA)
1 mandarin segmented
1 ½ tbsp raw honey
nutmeg to garnish

How to make it

Place all ingredients in a blender and mix well.
Top with shaved coconut.

My Body My Kitchen   Dr Kareem Samhouri

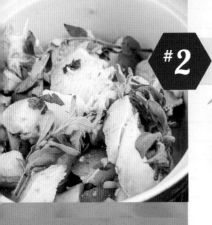

#2 Simple Chicken Stew

Preparation Time: 15 minutes *Cooking Time:* 35 minutes

This delicious, healthy meal will help you transition from the detox stage without becoming hungry. Free range, organic chicken is a healthy animal protein containing vitamin D that aids with calcium absorption and bone strengthening.

What's in it

2 tbsp avocado oil

2 large carrots, peeled and cut into 1-inch pieces

1 celery rib, chopped

sea salt to taste

freshly ground black pepper to taste

3 cloves garlic, minced

1 ½ lb chicken breasts, free-ranged organic suggested

3 sprigs thyme

1 bay leaf

¾ lb baby red-skinned potatoes, quartered

3 cups low-sodium chicken broth

2 tbsp parsley, chopped

How to make it

Heat oil in a large pot over medium heat.

Add carrots and celery. Cook until the vegetables are tender. About five minutes.

Add garlic and cook for 30 seconds.

Add chicken, thyme, bay leaf, potatoes and chicken broth. Simmer and cook for 15 minutes or until potatoes are tender and chicken is not pink.

Shred the chicken with a fork and return to the bowl.

Garnish with parsley.

Season with salt and pepper to taste.

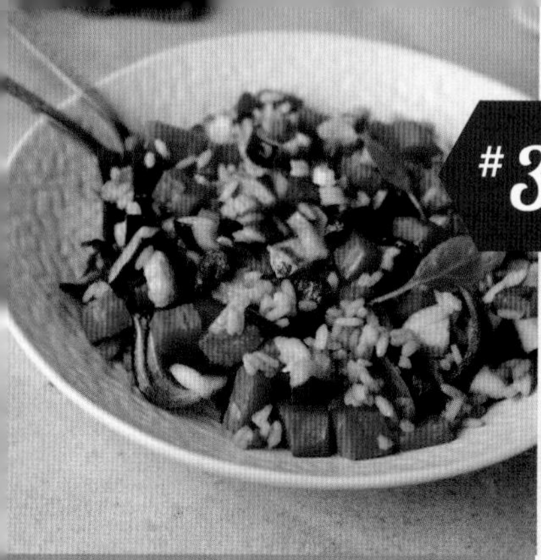

#3 Roasted Vegetable and Rice Salad

Preparation Time: 10 minutes   *Cooking Time:* 25 minutes

What's in it

1 cup cooked purple rice

2 small zucchini, chopped

1 medium carrot, chopped

1 small red onion, chopped

avocado oil to cover vegetables

2 small yellow summer squash, chopped

1 lemon, juiced

sea salt to taste

How to make it

Preheat oven to 300 ˚F. Lightly coat vegetables with avocado oil and roast until tender.

Cook the rice according to directions, or until all the water is absorbed.

Combine the vegetables with the rice in a large serving dish.

Serve warm with fresh lemon juice and sea salt.

Pair this warm and filling salad with a small piece of roasted chicken for a complete meal in a bowl.

My First Cookbook   Dr Kareem Samhouri

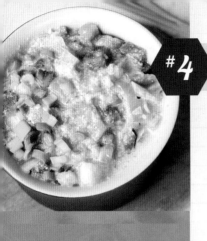

#4 Zucchini Chowder

Preparation Time: 15 minutes   *Cooking Time:* 40 minutes

This chowder has a bit of a kick, but is also smooth and creamy. Pair this with a big side salad for a fantastic lunch or dinner.

What's in it

3 tablespoons avocado oil
1 medium white onion, diced
2 large carrots, peeled and sliced
2 large celery ribs, chopped
2 large yellow zucchini diced
2 cloves garlic, minced
1 tbsp fresh ginger, peeled and minced
1 tsp ground turmeric
1 teaspoon ground cumin
4 cups low-sodium vegetable broth or chicken broth
½ cup almond milk
sea salt and freshly ground black pepper to taste
snipped chives, to garnish

How to make it

Heat avocado oil in a large stock pot.
Add the onion, carrots, and celery and cook until slightly tender
Add the garlic and ginger and cook for two more minutes.
Add in turmeric and cumin.
Pour in the vegetable broth and bring to a boil, lower and simmer with a lid for 20 minutes adding the diced zucchini for the last 3 minutes, remove from heat.
Using a handheld blender, blend half of the soup.
Leave some chunks of carrots and celery.
Pour in the almond milk and reheat.
Garnish with chives.

Tip: Chowder broth can be consumed non blended also.

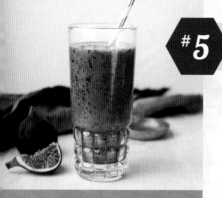

Fruit Juice Deluxe

Preparation Time: 5 minutes   *Cooking Time:* 3 minutes

What's in it

4 medium oranges

1 large fig

2 cups seedless black grapes

1 cup kiwi, peeled

1 tbsp raw honey

How to make it

Prepare all fruit and put through a juicer.

Stir in honey.

Serve immediately over ice optional.

Sometimes you just feel like a tasty juice. This mixture of fresh fruit is satisfying and full of essential vitamins and minerals to support a healthy transition from detox.

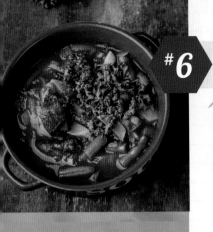

#6 Beef and Vegetable Soup

Preparation Time: 10 minutes   *Cooking Time:* 30 minutes

This recipe makes enough to feed six and is great for a family meal. Grass-fed beef is very nutrient dense and has as many omega-3's per serving as salmon.

What's in it

2 lbs ground beef - recommended grass-fed beef
¼ tsp cayenne pepper
1 cup diced potatoes
1 large leek, diced
2 carrots, diced
3 celery ribs, diced
4 cups beef broth
3 cups peeled and diced tomatoes
4 cups green cabbage, chopped
1 cup sliced green beans
fresh parsley
rice brand oil, to coat pan

How to make it

Warm a large stock pot over medium high heat and lighlty coat with rice bran oil, add the ground beef, Break meat down with a wooden spoon.
Brown the beef ensuring the meat is sealed.
Remove the beef from the pan and set aside.
Add the leek, potatoes, carrots and celery and a pinch of cayenne pepper to the pan.
Pour in the beef broth and tomatoes, and bring to a boil.
Add in cabbage, beans, and cooked beef, boil again.
Reduce the heat and simmer on low for ten minutes.
Serve with fresh minced parsley.

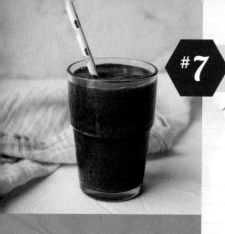

#7 Blueberry and Papaya Bliss

Preparation Time: 33 minutes   *Cooking Time:* 3 minutes

What's in it

- 1 cup diced papaya
- 1 cup frozen blueberries
- 1 cup coconut milk
- 1 tsp hemp seeds
- 1 tsp flax seeds

How to make it

Add all ingredients to a blender and blend until smooth.
Serve immediately.

Not only does this super smoothie offer a boatload of vitamins and minerals, the seeds also add omega 3 fatty acids, protein and fiber.

Dr Kareem Samhouri

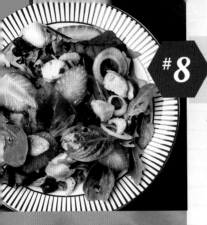

#8 Chicken and Strawberry Salad
(Tailored for Ectomorph)

Preparation Time: 10 minutes   *Cooking Time:* 5 minutes

50 minutes cooking time if including cooking Chicken

This colorful salad is full of flavor and health promoting ingredients. Tarragon triggers the stomach's natural digestive juices making it a powerful digestive aid. Plus, the balsamic vinegar adds just the right amount of zip.

What's in it

1 cup skinless chicken, roasted

2 whole fresh figs quartered

2 celery ribs, chopped

½ diced eschalot

2 tbsp dried cranberries

30gms or 2 tbsp of pistachio nuts

1 tbsp fresh tarragon, chopped

1 tbsp olive oil

1 tbsp balsamic vinegar

sea salt and pepper to taste

6 cups fresh salad greens

How to make it

Mix cranberries, celery, onion, and nuts together in a large bowl.

Combine tarragon, olive oil, vinegar, and salt and pepper.

Add the chicken to the greens along with the cranberry mixture and toss with the dressing.

Top with the figs and serve.

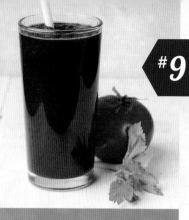

DIY Sweet Tomato Juice

Preparation Time: 10 minutes *Cooking Time:* 25 minutes

What's in it

> 4 cups tomatoes, diced
> ½ cup carrots, diced
> small sliver of beet
> 1 tbsp Worcestershire sauce
> ½ tsp sea salt
> ½ tsp black pepper
> 1 tsp raw honey
> ¼ cup baby spinach
> 1 tbsp parsley
> ½ cup of water

Lycopene, found in tomatoes, is a strong antioxidant that knocks out free radicals before they can cause cellular damage. The small sliver of beet not only helps with liver detoxification, but also gives this juice its naturally splendid sweet taste.

How to make it

Mix the tomatoes, carrots, beet, Worcestershire sauce, salt, pepper, honey, and ½ cup of water in a saucepan. Bring to a boil, reduce heat and simmer uncovered for 20 minutes.
Add the spinach and parsley and simmer covered for two minutes. Remove from heat and allow to cool .
Pour into blender. Blend until smooth and strain through a mesh sieve.
Serve cold.

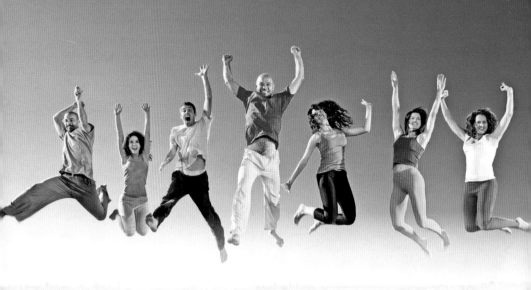

Lifestyle Recipes

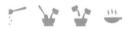

To insure good health: eat lightly, breathe deeply, live moderately, cultivate cheerfulness, and maintain an interest in life."

– William Londen

Body typing -- or using body morphology to determine your Body Type-- is a great way to provide more personalized recommendations surrounding health and nutrition. However, it's still a broad categorization, as each and every 'body' is unique. Your genetic makeup may be very similar -- or even the same -- as another person. However, the epigenetic variables -- or the choices you make throughout the day, and on a larger time scale -- affect which of your genes are being expressed at any given time.

New research shows that your genes are turning on or off every 2-3 minutes, which means you have an opportunity to optimize your health right now, regardless of the decision you made even a few minutes ago. That's super empowering, and it's really exciting to think of how you might look and feel when you turn 'on' your best genes.

Pretty cool, right?

Well, whether it's the foods you eat, where you live, the temperature in your house, how you think about -- and perceive -- the world, or how/when you move, you're having an impact on your genes. And what might be a superfood for one person may be a superfood for you when you feel great, and it may make you feel heavy and sluggish when you're already tired and cranky. Learn which foods agree with your body, and when, by experimenting with the guidelines of Body Type (ecto, endo, or mesomorph), and please recognize these are only guidelines.

Ultimately, the responsibility of knowing how and when to eat each type of food is on you. And we always advise you to have a conversation with your doctor and/or medical provider surrounding truly personalized nutrition and health. We believe in you, and we believe in your ability to transform the food you eat into pure, clean energy that makes you feel as though you're thriving throughout each and every day; while pleasing your taste buds at the same time.

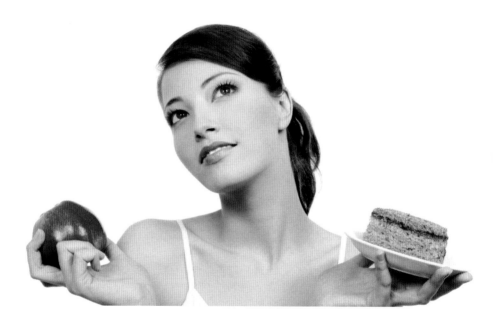

While we are unique, we have at least one thing in common: we are each designed to love the foods that are best for us; however, we must be free from eating all other foods for a period of weeks before our taste buds will completely adapt.

Living a healthy life and eating clean and nutritious food is not meant to be a pain. Instead, it is our hope that you will embrace all that eating a wholesome and clean diet has to offer. You will have so much energy, sleep great, and ward off damaging health conditions that could shorten your life. A healthy diet is the cornerstone of a long and vital life.

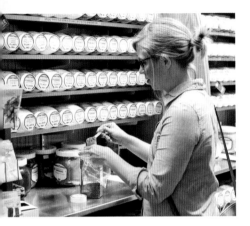

Enjoy your time in the kitchen, shop at your local farmers' markets, or grow your own food. Eating a wholesome diet is a rich and very rewarding experience that affects every area of your life.

As always, we encourage you to use only organic, raw, wild caught or grass fed ingredients.

ABBREVIATIONS

Endo: Suitable for endomorphs
Meso: Suitable for mesomorphs
Ecto: Suitable for ectomorphs

Endomorph Notes: If you are big-boned (short/stocky or big and tall): Lunch is your main meal of the day where animal protein and carbohydrates should be included. You should include a variety of meat sources and be heavy on green vegetables, always.

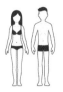

Main diet focus: moderate breakfast, main meal of the day lunch with a focus of no animal protein, sugars or carbohydrates after 4pm. Green vegetables, play a vital role also within an endomorph's daily intake requirements.

Foods to avoid: sugars, animal protein and heavy carbohydrates after 4 pm, (including whole fruit-based) and starches, processed meats.

Mesomorph Notes: If you are medium-boned and naturally athletic/strong for your body size: Eat 5x/day (with protein and vegetables), and (carbohydrates during day hours). Note that you can choose any recipe below that does not have animal protein and add a protein to it for a complete and well-balanced meal.

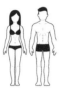

Main diet focus: animal-based proteins, vegetables, antioxidant-rich foods, eat until satisfied, not overeating but satisfied and comfortable.

Foods to avoid: inflammatory foods like excessive grain consumption, gluten and sugars after 4pm.

Ectomorph Notes: If you are average height to tall and thin-boned (or generally have a thinner frame). Eat warm foods, well-cooked meat 1-3 meals a day, lots of vegetables including root and high carbohydrate vegetables and pulses as well as orange and black fruits in color.

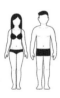

Main diet focus: variety of protein, fruits, and natural sugars like honey, vegetables and veggie juices, and smoothies, higher carbohydrate needs.

Foods to avoid: Undercooked meats, crisp vegetables, cold foods that require lots of energy for the body to warm, excessive inflammatory foods such as sugar and wheat (some gluten is ok, but limited), excessive protein intake (like eggs every day for breakfast, as an example)

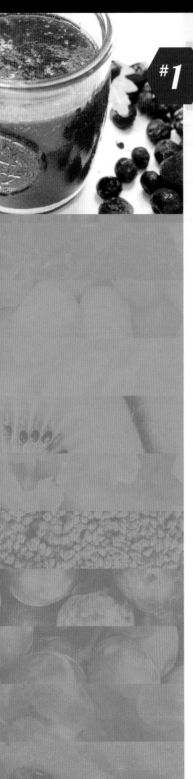

#1 Smoothie Super Booster (Endo, Meso, Ecto)

Preparation Time: 5 minutes   *Cooking Time:* 3 minutes

What's in it

- 1/8 cup or a handful of baby spinach leaves
- 1/8 cup shredded kale leaves - rib removed
- 3 large egg whites
- 2 tbsp hemp seeds
- 1/3 cup blueberries
- 1/2 cup fresh carrot juice
- 1/2 cup fresh blood orange juice
- 1 inch knob of fresh pressed ginger
- sprinkling of cinnamon

How to make it

Blend all ingredients in a high speed blender until smooth.
Top with a sprinkling of cinnamon.

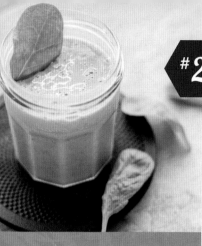

#2 Avocado and Papaya Smoothie (Endo, Meso)

Preparation Time: 5 minutes   **Cooking Time:** 3 minutes

What's in it

- ¼ avocado
- 1/3 cup fresh diced ripe papaya
- 1/8 cup or a handful of baby spinach leaves
- 2 arugula lettuce leaves
- 3 large egg whites
- 3/4 cup fresh carrot and mandarin juice
- 2 freshly pressed ginger juice
- 1/4 cup coconut water
- sprinkling of cinnamon or nutmeg

How to make it

Blend all ingredients except the coconut water in a high speed blender until thick and creamy.
Correct the consistency to your liking with the coconut water.
Enjoy immediately. Top with your choice of either cnnamon or nutmeg.

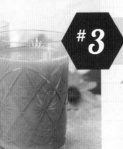

Morning, Light Cleanse (Ecto)

Preparation Time: 5 minutes　　*Cooking Time:* 3 minutes

What's in it

> 2 cups baby spinach
> 3 whole carrots
> 4 peeled blood oranges
> 2 peeled mandarins
> 2 inches knob of peeled ginger root
> ½ peeled lime
> 2 tbsp pressed unsweetened aloe vera juice

How to make it

> In a juicer, place the spinach in 3rd amounts at a time.
> Utilise the carrots to push through the spinach leaves.
> Juice all remaining ingredients.
> Lightly stir in aloe vera juice and consume.

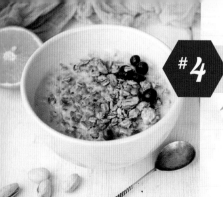

Steel Cut Oats (Endo, Meso, Ecto)

Preparation Time: 5 minutes   *Cooking Time:* 30 minutes

What's in it

1/2 cup steel cut oats
2/3 cup coconut water
1/2 cup almond milk

toppings

1/4 cup sheeps yogurt
1/4 cup blueberries
1/4 cup mandarin segments
1 tbsp raw Honey
2 tsp pistachio nuts
sprinkling of cinnamon

How to make it

Place oats, coconut water and almond milk in a medium saucepan, stir together and allow to stand for 10 minutes.
Place oats on a medium heat, stirring regularly until at a simmer.
Gently simmer for approximately 15 minutes, stirring regularly, until oats are cooked.
Additional coconut water can be used to obtain the desired consistency.
Add additional ingredients or preferred toppings.
Serve and enjoy.

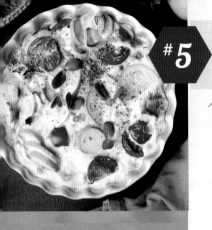

Goat's Milk, Zucchini and Tomato Frittata (Endo, Meso, Ecto)

Preparation Time: 10 minutes   **Cooking Time:** 30 minutes

If you like cheese but not all the calories, you'll love this quiche which calls for goat's cheese rather than your usual Swiss, brie or mozzarella. It has significantly less calories per ounce at just 75, and it's richer in essential nutrients, including vitamin A, vitamin B, riboflavin, calcium, iron, phosphorus, magnesium, and potassium.

What's in it

2 tbsp ghee butter

1 tbsp avocado oil

¼ leek sliced

1/4 cup diced yellow zucchini, (green can be used if out of season)

1/2 tsp Pink Himalayan salt

5 halved cherry tomatoes

1 whole eggs

3 large egg whites

1 cup raw goat's milk

1/3 cup crumbled goat cheese, shredded

oven paper

How to make it

Place butter and avocado oil in a pan and heat over medium. Once melted, add the leek cook for one minute, stirring frequently.

Add the zucchini, cook stirring frequently, until the zuchinni starts to soften, (do not overcook), remove from the heat and allow to slightly cool.

Beat all eggs with goats' milk and season with the Himalayan salt.

With a little ghee, grease the baking paper and place inside a frittata mould or suitable ovenware vessel.

Place the leek mixture into the mould.

Add the crumbled goat cheese and the tomatoes.

Pour the milk and egg mixture on top, ensuring the mixture reaches the bottom of the mould.

Slowly bake at 325F, the egg mixture in a moderate oven for approximately 15-20 mins, test that the egg is cooked by inserting a skewer, which when removed should come out clean.

Serve and enjoy.

Tip: Ectomorph can add some potatoes to their plate, maybe steamed potatoes with garlic and chives.

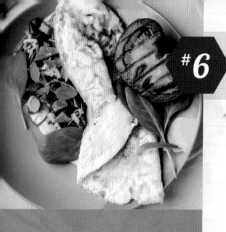

Farmhouse Spinach Omelette (Endo, Meso, Ecto)

Preparation Time: 8 minutes   **Cooking Time:** 3 minutes

Pre time increases to 20 mins if including cooking sweet potato

What's in it

3 large egg whites
1 whole egg
1/4 cup almond lilk
2 tsp snipped chives
pinch of pink or black himalayan salt

Filling

1 cups baby spinach
half leek, sliced
1/2 cup cooked and diced sweet potato (yam)
1 tbsp ghee butter
2 tsp avocado oil
1 whole vine ripened tomato, cut in half

How to make it

Beat eggs and whisk in the milk, season with the salt and snipped chives.

Warm 1/2 tablespoon of ghee and a little avocado oil in a saute pan.

Add leeks and gently cook until starting to soften, add the spinach and stir through, cook until spinach wilters, fold through the cooked warm sweet potato.

Place the halved cut tomato under a slow grill.

Place a omelet or suitable pan, onto warm with a little avocado oil, allow the pan / oil to heat up, discard the oil then add the remaining ghee, return to the stove,

Add the egg mixture to the pan and stir constantly until egg is softly cooked, remove from the heat and ensure the egg is spread to form an omelette.

Place the spinach mixture on the egg to one side and fold over the egg to create the omelette shape.

Turn the omelette onto a serving plate and add the grilled tomato.

Serve.

 Dr Kareem Samhouri

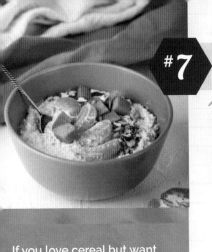

#7 Bran Muesli (Meso, Ecto)

Preparation Time: 5 minutes   *Cooking Time:* 15 minutes

If you love cereal but want something a bit heartier and more nutritious in the morning, this recipe is ideal.

What's in it

2 cups organic rice cereal bran flakes
1/4 cup almond milk
1/2 cup sheep or goat yogurt
2 tbsp raw honey
½ cup blueberries or fresh blackberries
½ cup mandarin segments or diced papaya
2 tbsp of linseed,sunflower and almond mix (LSA)

How to make it

Moisten the bran with the almond milk and allow to stand for 2 minutes,
Add the yogurt and fold together, allow to stand for 10 minutes.
Place the bran mixture in a serving bowl and top and decorate with the remaining ingredients.

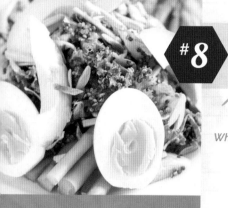

Hummus and Veggie Breakfast Bowl (Endo, Meso, Ecto)

🍴 **Preparation Time:** 12 minutes   🍲 **Cooking Time:** 10 minutes

What's in it - Makes for 4 (suitable alternative for 1 day a week)

1 tbsp avocado oil

1 pound asparagus, trim ends and cut into bite-sized pieces

2 cups kale leaves, finely shredded

3 cups brussels sprouts, shredded and un- cooked

1 ½ cups quinoa, cooked

½ cup hummus

1 avocado, peeled and sliced thin

4 poached eggs (optional)

2 tsp balsamic vinegar

2 tbsp olive oil

Garnishes: sunflower seeds, sliced almonds, toasted sesame seeds, crushed red pepper

How to make it

Heat oil in a large pan over medium-high heat.
Add asparagus and saute for 5 minutes, stirring occasionally until tender.
In a large mixing bowl, combine kale, balsamic vinegar, and oil. Rub the oil and vinegar into the kale for about 3 minutes, or until the leaves are dark and soft. Add the brussels sprouts, quinoa, and cooked asparagus. Toss together.
Divide the kale salad evenly between four bowls.
Top with a spoonful of hummus, avocado slices, egg (optional), and garnishes.
Serve immediately.

Tip: Ectomorphs, can warm through all of the vegetables, cook until kale and sprouts become soft.

This superfood breakfast bowl is tasty and provides an abundance of antioxidants, healthy fats, and protein. Brussels sprouts, kale, and asparagus are all naturally low in calories, high in fiber, and loaded with important nutrients. You'll get a big dose of protein too, thanks to the quinoa, eggs, and seeds.

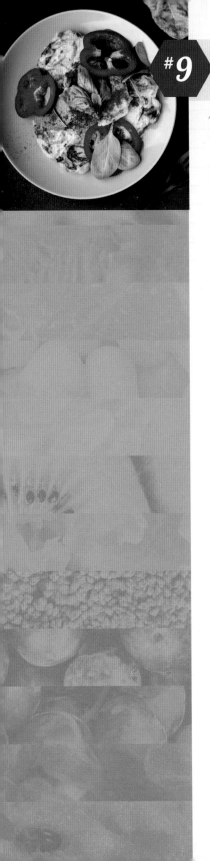

Bubble and Squeak... (Endo, Meso, Ecto)

 Preparation Time: 5 minutes 　*Cooking Time:* 15 minutes

Cooking time increases to 30 minutes if cooking potatoes

What's in it

1 tbsp ghee butter

1 cup sliced leek

1/2 cup cooked carrots

2 cups baby spinach

3 cups cooked mash potatoes

1 whole egg

2 tsp snipped chives

1 tsp grated nutmeg

pinch of Himalayan salt to taste

avocado oil for cooking

How to make it

Preheat the oven at 400 ˚F.

Slowly warm ghee over low heat in a medium sized pan.

Add leeks and cooked until softened

Add carrots then spinach turning to spinach wilters, remove from the heat.

Fold the mixture into the potatoes,

Whisk the egg and add to the mixture along with the chives, salt and grated nutmeg, fold through until all ingredients are well combined.

Form the potato mixture into your desired serving size portions

In a medium sized oven proof skillet, warm some avocado oil and place in the form potato mixture.

Allow cakes to cook to a golden color then turn.

Place the pan into the oven for an additional 3 minutes, checking not to over cook the cakes.

Remove from the oven and serve.

Tip: Add protein to the meal through quickly scrambling 3 large egg whites whisked with 1 whole egg and 1/8 of a cup of almond milk.

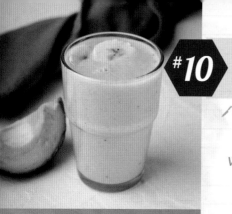

#10 Orange Whip Smoothie (Meso, Ecto)

Preparation Time: 5 minutes   **Cooking Time:** 3 minutes

What's in it

1 large banana, frozen
½ tsp vanilla extract
¾ cup fresh squeezed orange juice
½ cup coconut milk
1 medium avocado

optional: add 1 scoop vanilla whey protein powder

How to make it

Place all ingredients in a blender and blend until smooth.
Serve immediately.

Remember those incredibly yummy Dreamsicles? You know, the pale orange popsicles with creamy middles? Well this dish has a similar taste, but it's a lot healthier. Now you can enjoy the flavors of your childhood while feeding your body with the nutrition it needs to get you through the day.

Dr Kareem Samhouri

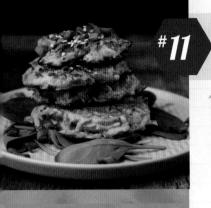

#11 Easy Vegetable Pancakes (Endo, Meso, Ecto)

Preparation Time: 10 minutes   *Cooking Time:* 16 minutes

Batch timing given for cooking

This recipe is not only easy to put together, but is also a whole new take on gluten-free pancakes. Get to grating, peeling, slicing, mincing and chopping, and in no time you'll have these fabulous vegetable pancakes that provide a great heart start in meeting your daily veggie needs.

What's in it

avocado oil to grease skillet
1 large yellow zucchini, grated
8 medium carrots, peeled and grated
1 bunch green onions, sliced
3 cloves garlic, minced
1/2 bunch fresh parsley, chopped
gluten-free pancake mix
salsa for topping

How to make it

Prepare the pancake mix according to directions, but use ¼ less water.
Fold in vegetables.
Warm a skillet over medium-high heat and brush it with avocado oil.
Scoop batter into skillet using a ⅓ cup measuring cup.
Cook until the outer edges are set. Flip and cook a few more minutes.
Sprinkle pancakes with salsa.

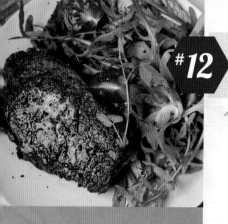

#12 Beef Breakfast Patty (Meso, Ecto)

Preparation Time: 15 minutes   **Cooking Time:** 8-12 minutes

Cooking time variance depending on degree of doneness.
Pre time includes forming patties.

These patty wraps are sure to become one of your breakfast favorites. While it may taste exactly like that store-bought stuff, the spices and other whole food ingredients in this recipe come together to create a much healthier dish without the added chemicals or preservatives.

What's in it

- 1 tbsp dried sage
- 3 diced eschallot bulbs
- ½ tsp red pepper flakes
- ½ tsp fennel seeds, crushed
- 1 lb beef mince
- 1 egg white
- salt and pepper, to taste
- rice bran oil, as needed

How to make it

Combine the sage, eschallot's, red pepper flakes, and fennel seeds.

Add the ground beef and mix.

Add the egg white and season with salt and pepper.

Wet your hands and divide the meat mixture into 8 equal portions, then flatten into patties that are ½ inch thick.

Heat 1 tbsp rice bran oil in a pan over medium-high heat. Add the patties, and fry until they are golden brown and cooked through. About 2 minutes per side. Serve and enjoy.

Meal pairing suggestions:

Enjoy your patty on a bed of sauteed wilted baby spinach with diced russet or yam potatoes, or alternatively a side of fresh fruit.

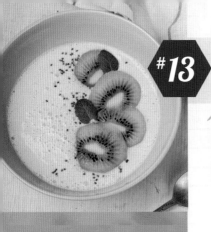

#13 Lemon Yogurt Smoothie Soup (Endo, Meso, Ecto)

Preparation Time: 5 minutes   *Cooking Time:* 5 minutes

What's in it

1/2 cup goat's milk yogurt
1/2 cup coconut milk
1 tbsp honey
1/2-inch piece fresh ginger, peeled
1/2 tsp freshly grated lemon zest
1/2 tsp ground turmeric
1/2 tsp chia seeds
1/2 cup pomegranate seeds
½ cup diced kiwi fruit

How to make it

Put all ingredients except the fruit, in a blender and blend on high speed until smooth and creamy. Place in a serving bowl and decorate with the fruit.

This "lemonlicious" smoothie soup proves that healthy food doesn't have to taste bland and uninteresting. Smoothies are ideal for breakfast - they only take minutes to make and can keep you full all morning. The coconut milk in this recipe adds healthy, filling fats to keep you satisfied longer, and the ginger and turmeric help boost energy. You'll also get a good dose of amino acids thanks to the chia seeds.

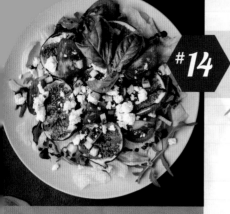

#14 Fig and Goat Crumble (Endo, Meso, Ecto)

Preparation Time: 10 minutes   **Cooking Time:** 5 minutes

Pair this warm and filling salad with a small piece of roasted chicken for a complete meal in a bowl.

What's in it

- 3 fresh figs halved
- 2 tbsp goats cheese crumble
- 8 cherry tomatoes
- 1 diced eschallot bulb
- 1/2 cup arugula leaves
- 1 tbsp avocado oil
- 1 tbsp balsamic vinegar
- 1 tbsp apple cider vinegar
- ½ cup diced skinned cucumber
- ½ cup diced celery
- 1 tbsp snipped chives or fresh basil leaves

How to make it

In a small saute pan, heat a little avocado oil, add the cherry tomatoes and slowly cook until the first pop.
Lightly rinse the arugula leafs and pat dry, lay the leaves on the base of a serving plate or bowl.
Cut the figs and evenly place on the lettuce.
Place the cucumber, celery, eschallots, apple cider and balsamic vinegar in a bowl and combine together.
Sprinkle the marinated mix over the figs.
Top with the blistered tomatoes and crumble on the goats cheese.
Garnish with snipped chives or basil.

Dr Kareem Samhouri

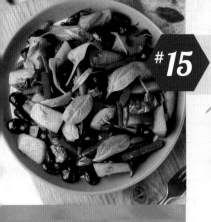

Breakfast Stir Fry (Endo, Meso, Ecto)

🍴 **Preparation Time:** 20 minutes   ☕ **Cooking Time:** 10 minutes

Prep time includes cooking potatoes.

Stir-fry is one of the easiest meals to put together. It only takes minutes, and if you use the right ingredients, it's an especially nutritious dish as well. While you might think stir-fry is just a dinner meal, why not change things up and enjoy some at breakfast? This recipe includes a rainbow of brightly colored vegetables along with black beans for an added boost of protein. With diced potatoes included as well, you won't have to worry about mid-morning hunger pangs.

What's in it

½ onion, chopped

1 carrot, sliced thinly

½ bell pepper, sliced

½ red pepper, sliced

1 cup cooked potatoes, diced

½ cup black beans, cooked

1 jalapeno, sliced

2 tbsp liquid aminos, optional

2/3 cup baby spinach

1 ½ cups fresh asparagus, halfed

1 tbsp avocado oil

1/3 cup vegetable stock

How to make it

Warm pan and coat with oil.

Add onion and carrot to a large skillet and cook for a few minutes, covered.

Add bell pepper and red pepper and stir. Cook for a few minutes more. If vegetables are sticking, put a little water in the pan.

Add cooked potatoes, beans, and jalapeno. Add vegetable stock and bring to a simmer. Cook for a few more minutes.

Once the potatoes are warmed, add aminos and stir again.

Add spinach and asparagus and put lid on skillet, do not stir. Cook for about 5 more minutes.

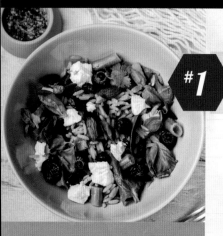

#1

Superfood Salad (Endo, Meso, Ecto)

Preparation Time: 20 minutes   *Cooking Time:* 5 minutes
Prep time includes rice.

Pair this warm and filling salad with a small piece of roasted chicken for a complete meal in a bowl.

What's in it

For the dressing

> 1/4 cup olive oil
>
> 1/4 cup honey
>
> 1/4 cup apple cider vinegar
>
> 2 tsp dijon mustard
>
> ¾ tsp Himalayan sea salt
>
> ¾ tsp black pepper

For the salad

> 2 cups cooked warm purple rice
>
> 2 cups fresh spinach
>
> 1 cup blueberries
>
> 1 cup crumbled feta
>
> ½ cup dried cranberries
>
> ¾ cup goat's cheese, shaved
>
> 2 cups cooked warm diced green beans
>
> ½ cup sliced almonds
>
> 1/4 cup fresh basil or cilantro, finely chopped

How to make it

Dressing

> Place all ingredients in a small jar with a lid.
> Put the lid on and shake vigorously until all ingredients combine.

Salad

> Add all ingredients in order to a large mixing bowl.
> Drizzle with dressing and toss.

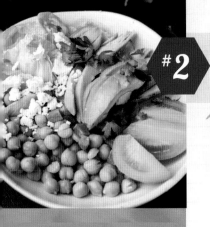

#2

Chickpea Salad Bowl
(Endo, Meso, Ecto)

Preparation Time: 25 minutes　　*Cooking Time:* 5 minutes
Prep time includes cooking chicken and sweet potatoes.

This salad is based on one of nature's true wonder foods, chickpeas. They're loaded with protein at 16 grams per cup and are also a rich source of fiber, essential for maintaining a healthy digestive system and keeping you full longer. With the chicken and sweet ripe papaya, you'll feel as if you're at a summer picnic every time you enjoy this salad.

What's in it

2 large romaine hearts, washed and chopped

1 cup chicken breast, pulled and cooked (keep warm)

1 15.5 oz can chickpeas, rinsed and drained

1 cup grape tomatoes, sliced in half

3/4 cup diced papaya

1/4 cup crumbled goat cheese

1 cup diced cooked and warm sweet potatoes

1/3 cup cilantro, washed and chopped

1 small avocado, diced

How to make it

Add lettuce to a large bowl and top with all other ingredients except avocado. Toss lightly.
Place salad in serving bowls and top with diced avocado.

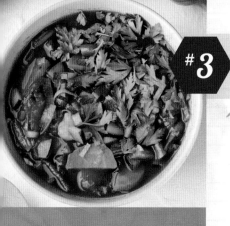

#3 Special Garden Soup (Endo, Meso, Ecto)

Preparation Time: 20 minutes   *Cooking Time:* 40 minutes

What's in it

4 tbsp rice bran oil

2 cups chopped leeks,

2 tbsp garlic, minced

Himalayan sea salt, to taste

cracked black pepper, to taste

2 cups carrots, peeled and chopped into rounds

2 cups potatoes, peeled and diced

2 cups green beans, broken into ¾-inch pieces

8 cups vegetable broth

4 cups tomatoes, peeled, deseeded, and chopped

1 cup diced yellow zucchini

¼ cup packed parsley leaves, chopped

2 tsp freshly squeezed lemon juice

How to make it

Heat rice bran oil in a large stockpot over medium-low heat.

When hot, add leeks, garlic, and salt and cook about 2 minutes.

Add carrots, potatoes, and green beans. Cook for 5 more minutes, stir occasionally.

Add the broth and bring the soup to a simmer.

Add tomatoes, zucchini and black pepper. Reduce the heat to low, cover and cook until vegetables are tender. About 25 minutes.

Remove from heat and add parsley and lemon juice. Season with salt and pepper to taste.

Want to use the bounty of vegetables your garden has produced? This soup is a great way to do just that, or use this recipe as inspiration to start your own garden. Not only is this soup incredibly tasty, but it has such an array of colorful vegetables that you know it's going to pack a nutritional punch as well.

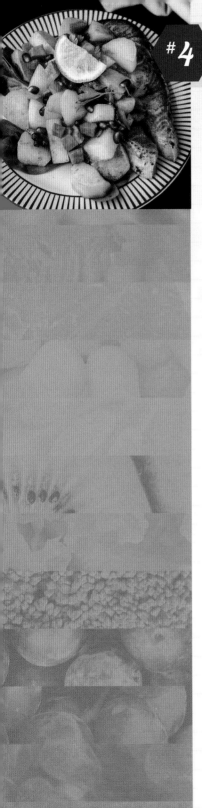

Summer Salmon with a Salsa Sensation (Endo, Meso, Ecto)

 # 4

Preparation Time: 10 minutes

Cooking Time: 30 minutes
Cooking time includes potatoes.

What's in it

5 to 6 oz salmon fillet skin on
1 tbsp rice bran oil
1 cup diced cooked potatoes (keep warm)
½ cup warm asparagus spears
¼ cup pomegranate seeds
1 cup diced papaya
½ tsp Himalayan salt
¼ tsp fine cracked black pepper
¼ cup cilantro leaves
¼ tsp red pepper flakes or fresh sliced red chili
1 tbsp apple cider vinegar
¼ cup diced bell peppers
1 tsp lime juice
1 tsp chopped mint

How to make it

Place potatoes to cook and water for the asparagus, prepare all other ingredients.

When potatoes are ¾'s cooked, heat a small skillet pan and warm the oil.

Place the salmon fillet skin down into the pan and allow to stand and cook, shake pan at times to ensure the fillet isn't sticking, leave fillet skin down until golden brown (2-3 mins approx), once colored turn the fillet over and continue to cook for an additional one minute, remove from heat and allow to rest.

Place the asparagus on to cook.

Once potatoes are cooked, strain off all of the cooking liquid and then leave the potatoes to stand and release steam.

In a separate bowl place the papaya, pomegranate, chili, bell peppers and mint leaves and lightly mix together, then add the cooked asparagus.

Pour the vinegar onto the potatoes and add to the papaya bowl, ensure to gently fold the ingredients together

Place an amount of the combined potato mix in the centre of the serving plate.

Place the warm salmon fillet on top, then another amount of the combined potato mix on top of the salmon, allow the volume of the mix to fall down.

Sprinkle the meal with the fresh lime juice and cilantro leaves, serve.

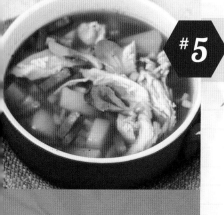

Comfort Chicken Soup (Endo, Meso, Ecto)

Preparation Time: 10 minutes *Cooking Time:* 50 minutes

What's in it

- 3 lb chicken
- 4 cups chicken broth
- 2 cups cooked potatoes
- 6 cups water
- ½ cup onion, chopped
- 1 tsp fresh ginger, grated
- 3-4 cups carrots, chopped
- 2-3 cups celery, chopped
- 6-8 garlic cloves, minced
- 1 tsp ground turmeric
- ½ tbsp basil
- ½ tbsp parsley
- 3 tbsp coconut aminos
- 1 tsp Himalayan salt, or to taste
- ¼ tsp black pepper, or to taste

There are few things better on a cold day, or when you're feeling under the weather, than chicken soup. This recipe contains everything you need to help get that health back on track. Ginger is known for its ability to cleanse the body of toxins by stimulating sweating, digestion, and circulation. While garlic and turmeric are fabulous spices that can help boost your immune system.

How to make it

Add chicken to a large soup pot filled with 6 cups of water. Bring to a boil and reduce the heat and simmer for about 30 minutes or until fully cooked. Set aside.
Add broth and 6 cups of water that the chicken was cooked in to a large soup pot. Add in onions, ginger, carrots, celery, garlic, and turmeric. Bring to a boil, reduce heat, cover and cook for about 10 minutes. While the broth and vegetables are cooking. Shred the cooled chicken with a fork and add it along with the cooked potatoes, basil, parsley, salt and pepper, and coconut aminos to the pot.
Bring the soup to a boil, lower the heat, cover and simmer until the vegetables are tender.
Add additional herbs if desired.

 Dr Kareem Samhouri

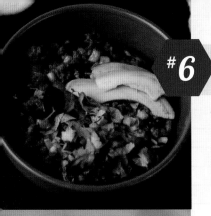

#6 Chili Beef (Endo, Meso, Ecto)

Preparation Time: 15 minutes   *Cooking Time:* 60 minutes

What's in it

Do you like a spicy, hearty chili? It's hard to beat this recipe when it comes to nutrition and taste. It's filled with a variety of beans that offer lots of healthy, filling fiber, though the bison is the real star. Healthier than grass-fed beef and richer in flavor, it has less calories and fat and is an excellent source of lean protein.

3 poblano peppers, seeded and diced

2 medium onions, diced

2 tsp rice bran oil

2 lbs lean ground beef or bison

6 tbsp chili powder

1 tsp ground coriander

1 tsp ground cumin

1 tsp sea salt

1 tsp cayenne pepper

3 cloves garlic, minced

1 14.5 oz can whole fire-roasted tomatoes, crushed

1 15.5 oz can black beans, drained and rinsed

1 15.5 oz can red kidney beans, drained and rinsed

1 15.5 oz can white hominy, drained and rinsed

1 bunch cilantro leaves

1 red onion, diced finely

2 avocados, sliced

4 cups water

How to make it

Heat 1 tsp oil in a large pot over medium heat.

Add ground meat and cook until brown. Remove meat from the pot and set aside.

Add 1 tsp oil to the same pot along with poblano peppers and onion. Cook until they begin to brown, about 5 minutes.

Add chili powder, coriander, cumin, salt, cayenne pepper, and garlic. Cook until the spices are fragrant.

Add the tomatoes with juice and bring to a simmer for about 2 minutes. Put the cooked meat, beans, and 4 cups water into the pot. Bring to a boil, reduce heat, cover and simmer until thick, about 45 minutes.

Season with salt and pepper.

Top with diced red onion, cilantro and avocado.

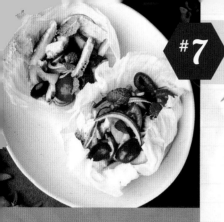

Greek Baked Chicken in Cos Pockets (Endo, Meso, Ecto)

Preparation Time: 30 minutes *Cooking Time:* 15 minutes

Prep time includes marination time for chicken.

Filled with the flavors of the Mediterranean, including olives, and juicy grape tomatoes. You may want to make extra for an easy office lunch.

What's in it

- 1 lb chicken breast
- ½ lemon, juiced
- 6 tbsp extra-virgin olive oil, divided
- 1 tsp dried oregano
- 3 small garlic cloves, minced and divided
- sea salt to taste
- black pepper to taste
- 1 cucumber, seeded, quartered, and sliced thinly
- ½ cup diced celery
- 1/2 pt. yellow grape tomatoes, cut in half lengthwise
- 1/2 pt. red grape tomatoes, cut in half lengthwise
- 1/2 red onion, sliced thin into half moons
- 1/4 cup fresh mint, chopped
- 1 cup artichoke quarters
- 1/4 cup pitted Kalamata olives, cut in half
- 2 tbsp red wine vinegar
- 8 whole wash romaine lettuce leaves

How to make it

In a small bowl combine lemon juice, 2 tbsp olive oil, oregano, and 2 garlic cloves for marinade.

Place chicken breasts in a shallow baking dish, and pour marinade over them. Marinate for 15 minutes.

Bake the chicken at 350 ˚F until cooked through, ensuring to check often to prevent over coloring, then slice thinly.

Combine cucumber, tomatoes, celery, artichokes, red onion, olives and mint in a large bowl. Toss.

Whisk together red wine vinegar and garlic clove. Add 4 tablespoons olive oil and whisk well. Add salt and pepper, drizzle over vegetable salad and toss lightly.

Layer the mixture and chicken into the romaine lettuce leaves.

Tip: Add an accompaniment of a warm savoury purple rice portion or a warm yam to your meal.

Dr Kareem Samhouri

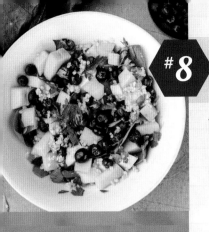

#8 Quinoa Fruit Salad (Endo, Meso, Ecto)

Preparation Time: 10 minutes   *Cooking Time:* 10 minutes

What's in it

This salad is another great way to use quinoa. It not only adds a nice crunch to a fruit salad, but also provides that all-important protein and all nine essential amino acids. The fabulous mix of fruit and vegetables ensures that it's antioxidant packed too. The healthy fat from the avocado means you'll be keeping those hunger pangs at bay and your metabolism burning at its max.

For the dressing
¼ cup fresh lime juice
1 ½ tsp honey
1 tsp apple cider vinegar
1/8 tsp ginger
pinch of salt, to taste

For the salad
3/4 cup quinoa
6 cups organic baby spinach, diced
⅓ cup red onion, dice
1 cup blueberries
1 ripe mango, diced
¼ cup cilantro, chopped
½ ripe avocado, diced

How to make it

Cook quinoa according to directions.
For the dressing, combine lime juice, honey, apple cider vinegar, ginger, and a pinch of salt in a medium bowl. Whisk together until combined. Set aside.
Combine spinach, red onion, blueberries, mango, cilantro, and avocado to the quinoa and mix gently with a wooden spoon.
Drizzle dressing on top and mix well.

Tip: Ideal protein to add could be salmon, trout, or lamb fillets.

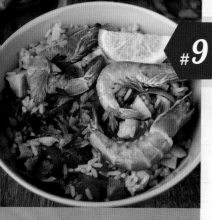

Seafood Paella (Endo, Meso, Ecto)

Preparation Time: 15 minutes   *Cooking Time:* 20 minutes

What's in it

- 1 cup purple rice
- 2 diced eschallot bulbs
- 1 cup mixed diced bell peppers
- 4 cloves garlic, chopped
- 1 diced fennel bulb
- 1 cup finely diced carrots
- ½ cup diced celery
- ½ tsp chili flakes (optional)
- 2 cups organic fish or chicken stock
- 3 prawns
- ½ cup cod fillet strips
- 1 lime
- freshly chopped cilantro, to garnish
- 1/2 tbsp ghee butter
- baking paper
- 2 tbsp avocado oil

How to make it

Pre-heat the oven at 425 °F.

Heat the avocado oil in a oven proof lidded pan.

Add the eschallots, garlic and carrots to the pan, cook until eschallots start to soften.

Add the rice, stir completely the rice through, to ensure the rice becomes coated with the oil.

Add the celery, fennel, chili and stir through.

Add the stock to just cover the rice, stir through to allow the stock to cover everything.

Return to a simmering point, add the cod and prawn pieces and cover fully with greased (ghee) baking paper, lid and place in the oven, for approximately 7 minutes.

Check occasionally on the rice and the liquid, add more liquid if required.

When rice is cooked, serve either in the baking pan or on a serving plate,

Squeeze some lime juice over the rice and top with the cilantro leaves, serve.

Dr Kareem Samhouri

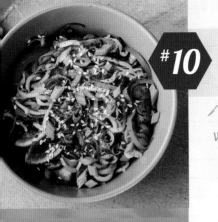

#10 Hot Veggie Noodle Bowl (Endo, Meso, Ecto)

Preparation Time: 15 minutes   *Cooking Time:* 10 minutes

What's in it

8 oz yellow and green zucchini strips / noodles

½ cup carrot strips

1 tbsp lime zest, freshly grated

2 tbsp lime juice

3 tbsp liquid aminos

1/2 tbsp chili flakes

½ tbsp crushed-garlic

1 tbsp coconut sugar / coconut nectar crystals

2 tbsp coconut oil

4 large eggs, beaten

3 cups shitake mushroom caps, sliced

2 red peppers, sliced

3 cups finely shredded napa green cabbage

1 bunch scallions, sliced and divided

Many of us lived on Ramen noodles in our college years, which may be why we get those occasional cravings that take us back to another time. Unfortunately, it's not the healthiest choice, but there are ways to satisfy those desires, allowing us to enjoy the taste and comfort without the guilt. While your craving will be indulged, you'll still be supporting your good health.

How to make it

Make the vegetable noodles on a spiralizer or similar. Cook the carrot noodle strips, maintaining a little firmness bite still to the carrots, cool immediately.

Mix, the lime zest and juice, aminos, chili,garlic and coconut sugar in a small bowl. Set aside.

Heat a 14-inch flat bottom wok over high heat. Add 1 teaspoon oil and swirl to coat the pan. Add eggs and tilt the wok to create an omelet. Cook until set. Turn the omelet over and cook 30 seconds more. Cut the omelet into thin strips. Set aside.

Add another tablespoon of oil along with mushrooms and bell pepper to the wok. Stir fry for 2 minutes. Add cabbage, zucchini, carrots and half of the scallions and cook until vegetables are tender.

Add the chile-lime sauce, Toss

Add the egg strips and stir-fry until heated through. Sprinkle with scallions.

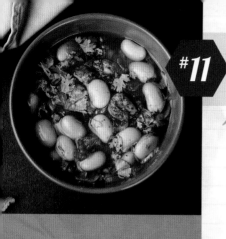

Zesty Lupini Bean Soup (Endo, Meso, Ecto)

Preparation Time: 5minutes   *Cooking Time:* 15 minutes

What's in it

1 tbsp avocado oil
1 small yellow onion, chopped
1 tbsp chili powder
1 tsp ground cumin
2 15-oz cans lupini, rinsed
3 cups water
½ cup salsa
½ tsp sea salt
1 tbsp lime juice
2 tbsp fresh cilantro

Beans of all types, including Lupini beans, are packed with satisfying fiber to keep you feeling full longer while also supporting heart health. They contain lots of protein and a number of essential nutrients, like calcium, potassium, and magnesium. With the added spices, this zesty soup is sure to please and can help rev up your metabolism too.

How to make it

Heat oil in a large saucepan over medium heat. Add the onion and cook until it begins to soften.
Add chili powder and cumin and cook for 1 minute. Keep stirring. Add the beans, water, salsa, and salt and bring to a boil. Reduce the heat and simmer for about 10 minutes.
Remove from heat and add the lime juice.
Serve with cilantro garnish.

Optional - Place the soup into a blender and blend until smooth. Return to the saucepan to reheat.

Tip: Add strips of poached chicken to increase the protein.

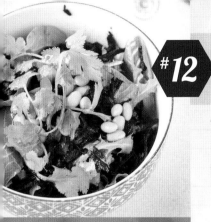

#12 All That Green Salad (Endo)

Preparation Time: 10 minutes   *Cooking Time:* 3 minutes

What's in it

2 cups mixed salad greens
1 cup shelled edamame, thawed
½ medium raw beet, peeled and shredded

For the dressing

1 tbsp red wine vinegar
1 tbsp fresh cilantro, chopped
2 tsp extra-virgin olive oil
sea salt to taste
black pepper to taste

How to make it

Arrange the vegetables on a large plate.
Whisk vinegar, cilantro, olive oil, and salt and pepper in a small bowl. Drizzle on salad and enjoy.

Green is a fabulous color when it comes to your health; just about any type of salad green can be considered a superfood. With this recipe, you can choose your favorites. From arugula with its rich, peppery flavor, to kale with leaves that are jam-packed with vitamins and minerals. Toss in some edamame, and you've even got your protein. 1 cup contains 17 grams.

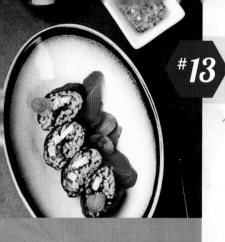

Nori Rolls with Sweet Turkey (Endo, Meso, Ecto)

🖊 *Preparation Time:* 25 minutes   🍲 *Cooking Time:* 10 minutes

If you're a fan of Sushi rolls, you'll love this dish. By using purple rice instead of white, you'll be getting high amounts of manganese, selenium, magnesium, phosphorus and B vitamins along with a substantial amount of fiber and protein per serving.

What's in it

For the sauce

- 1½ tsp sesame oil
- 1½ tsp apple cider vinegar
- 1 tsp raw honey
- 1 tsp liquid aminos
- 1 tsp water
- ½ tsp garlic, minced
- ¼ tsp red pepper flakes

For the salad

- 3 nori sheets
- 1 cup cooked purple rice
- ½ cup shaved turkey breast
- ¼ cup dried cranberries
- ¼ cup diced water chestnuts
- ¼ cup avocado, sliced
- fresh cilantro leaves to taste
- fresh mint leaves to taste
- sushi pink pickled ginger to taste

How to make it

Combine the sauce ingredients in a small bowl and whisk until smooth.

Lay out all of the ingredients across the 3 sheets of nori.

Add cilantro, mint and sushi ginger to taste.

Role and allow to sit for 5 mins on a board with the end of the nori roll facing down.

Serve.

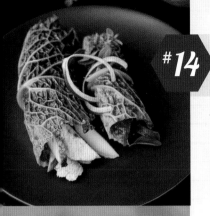

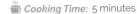

#14 Roasted Turkey Kale Lunch Wraps (Meso, Endo)

Preparation Time: 10 minutes   *Cooking Time:* 5 minutes

This recipe is a great way to use that leftover Thanksgiving turkey. In fact, you could call it a Thanksgiving meal wrap, minus the gravy and potatoes. The cranberry sauce adds a wonderful touch, bringing all those flavors together, and the kale leaves pack a fantastic nutritional punch.

What's in it

1 tbsp low sugar cranberry sauce
1 tbsp Dijon mustard
3 medium lacinato kale leaves
3 slices roasted turkey slices
6 slices red onion
1 ripe pear, cut into 9 thin slices

How to make it

Combine the cranberry sauce and mustard in a small bowl. Spread on kale leaves.
Top each leaf with a slice of turkey, 2 slices of red onion and 3 slices of pear.
Roll each leaf like a wrap.

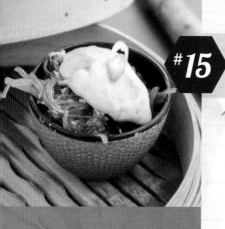

Wakame Seaweed Salad with Sea Iron (Endo, Meso, Ecto)

🖋 **Preparation Time:** 35 minutes   🍲 **Cooking Time:** 3 minutes

What's in it

- 6 fresh oyster in half shell
- 2 cups dried wakame seaweed
- 2 shallots finely sliced (optional)
- 1 tsp apple cider vinegar
- 1 tsp sesame oil
- 1 tsp yuzu juice
- 1 tsp mirin
- 1 tsp sesame seeds (white or black)

Optional Additions

- Pinch cayenne pepper or finely sliced red chili (to taste)
- grated fresh root ginger

How to make it

Place the dried seaweed in a large bowl, cover with luke warm water until soft and tender (up to 20 mins).

While the seaweed is soaking, prepare the dressing, combine the vinegar, oil, yuzu and mirin in a bowl. Add the ginger at this point also if using.

Drain the seaweed, pat the seaweed dry, then cut into strips.

Place in a bowl and pour over the dressing.

Mix well and allow to stand for 10 mins, turn every few minutes.

Loosen the oysters from their shells. Rinse the oysters, ensure to check the shell an underlying area of the oyster.

Fill each oyster shell with the seaweed salad.

Place the oysters back on top.

Decorate with a little more salad and sesame seeds.

Serve.

Tip: If you don't like oysters, replace with any fish or even avocado.

And if you need some carbohydrates, then add a warm rice salad, double up the seaweed dressing to pour over the rice, and add a few more shallots on the rice as well.

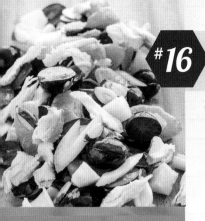

#16 Chicken Fruit Salad (Endo, Meso)

Preparation Time: 20 minutes
Prep time includes cooking chicken.

Cooking Time: 5 minutes

While a fruit salad isn't very filling on its own, combine it with chicken and you have a wonderfully refreshing salad that will keep you going all afternoon. The pineapple, grapes and clementine are perfectly combined to adds lots of juicy flavor, so you won't be missing out on taste either.

What's in it

- ¼ cup toasted almonds, chopped
- 2 cups chicken breasts, cooked and chopped
- 2 cups seedless red and green grapes, cut in half
- 2 celery ribs, chopped
- 2 cups clementine pieces
- 1 cup fresh pineapple, chopped
- ¼ tsp sea salt
- ¼ tsp black pepper
- 2 tsp balsamic vinegar
- 2 tbsp olive oil

How to make it

Toss the ingredients together in a bowl.
Combine balsamic vinegar and olive oil.
Sprinkle with salt and pepper and top with balsamic vinegar and olive oil mixture.

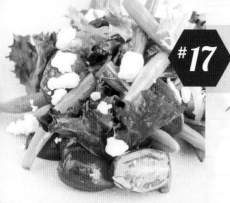

#17 Tomato and Basil Salad with Goat Cheese (Endo, Meso)

Preparation Time: 10 minutes   *Cooking Time:* 35 minutes

What's in it

1 cup cherry tomatoes, cut in half
½ cup fresh basil, torn
¼ cup goat's cheese, crumbled
½ cup artichoke quarters
1 cup cooked green beans
1 garlic clove, minced
1 tbsp olive oil
½ tbsp balsamic vinegar
¼ tsp himalayan salt
¼ tsp black pepper
¼ tsp oregano
lettuce (cos / arugula / spinach)

This salad may be simple, but it's a true Mediterranean delight, with goat cheese, cherry tomatoes, and fresh basil helping to bring it all together. When you don't have a lot of prep time available, it may become your go-to salad. All you have to do is toss the ingredients together and let it chill for a while.

How to make it

Combine all ingredients, except the goats cheese and let sit for about 30 minutes.
Serve over a bed of lettuce and sprinkle over the goat's cheese.

Dr Kareem Samhouri

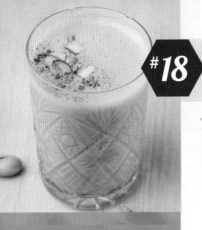

#18 Super Superfood Smoothie (Endo, Meso, Ecto)

Preparation Time: 20 minutes   *Cooking Time:* 3 minutes

What's in it

1/2 cup chopped carrots, steamed and cooled if you do not have a high-power blender

1/2 cup chopped sweet potatoes, steamed and cooled if you do not have a high-power blender

1/2 cup banana, sliced and frozen

1 cup kefir

1/4 cup frozen, diced pineapple

2 tbsp pistachio

1/4 tsp cinnamon

pinch nutmeg

How to make it

If you have a high-powered blender there is no need to steam carrots and sweet potato. Otherwise, steam them for a few minutes to soften.

Place all ingredients into the blender and blend until smooth.

Smoothies are an easy way to get the nutrition you need all packed into an easy on-the-go glass. With this recipe, you'll get lots of beta carotene, thanks to the carrots and sweet potatoes, along with the tropical flavors of pineapple, coconut, and banana. The coconut milk contains healthy fats that are sure to keep you satisfied so you won't be reaching for junk just a couple of hours later.

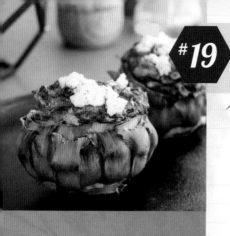

#19 Baked Artichokes (Endo, Meso, Ecto)

🔪 **Preparation Time:** 15 minutes 🍲 **Cooking Time:** 30 minutes

What's in it

6 fresh artichokes
juice of 1 lemon
2 tsp avocado oil
2 eschallots, finely diced
2 tsp finely chopped flat leaf parsley
½ cup crumbled sheep cheese
2 cups baby spinach
1 tsp crushed garlic
6 peeled and chopped plum tomatoes
½ cup tomato juice
1 tbsp apple cider vinegar
pinch pink Himalayan salt
freshly chopped basil, garnish
balsamic vinegar drizzle
black pepper to taste

How to make it

Preheat an oven at 300 °F
In a saucepan, heat the avocado oil, add the eschallots, garlic and saute for 1 minute.
Add the chopped tomatoes and juice, along with the vinegar.
Simmer on stove, stirring occasionally until liquid has reduced by ¼, then set a side.
Wash the artichokes and trim about 1 inch from the top, remove the tough outer leaves and trim the stem. With a spoon carefully remove the centre (looks like fine hairs).
Place the prepared artichokes in water with the lemon juice.
Return the tomato sauce to the stove and when warm add the baby spinach. Cook until spinach binds with the sauce and remove from the heat.
Add the sheep's cheese and allow to blend
Remove the artichokes from the water and drain them well.
With a spoon fill the artichokes with the filling and arrange the artichokes in a baking dish.
Cover and baked for 20 mins, then uncover and bake for an additional five minutes.
Arrange the artichokes in a large bowl and top with any left over filling and pan juices.
Drizzle with some balsamic vinegar and sprinkle with basil, parsley and finely cracked black pepper to taste, serve.

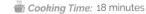

#1

Wrapped Fish with Fennel
(Meso, Ecto)

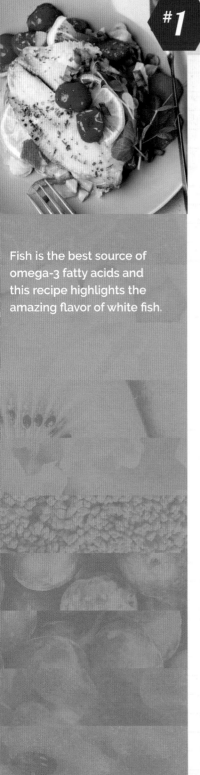

Fish is the best source of omega-3 fatty acids and this recipe highlights the amazing flavor of white fish.

🍴 *Preparation Time:* 20 minutes   ☕ *Cooking Time:* 18 minutes

What's in it

4 portions - 5 to 6 oz skinless fish serving per portion - Asian sea bass, barramundi, sole, cod, salmon or trout.
1 shallots , sliced
1 carrots, finely sliced
1 celery ribs, sliced
12 cherry tomatoes, halved
1 cup sliced fennel
1 garlic cloves, minced
1/4 tsp Pink Himalayan sea salt
1/4 tsp fine cracked black pepper
1 tbsp fresh herbs (combine minced parsley, dill, basil)
4 slices of lemon
¼ cup coconut water
baking paper
1/2 tbsp ghee butter
sushi pickled ginger garnish
snipped chives garnish

How to make it

Preheat oven to 350 ˚F.
Ensure fish fillet are prepared and clean,
Prepare all other ingredients,
Cut baking paper into 11 inches x 11 inches square, grease lightly in the center with ghee.
On the ghee base, evenly spread and sprinkle the garlic, carrots, celery, shallots and fennel, over 4 equal portions.
Then place one fish fillet on top of each, Sprinkle with salt and pepper, tomatoes and herbs, lay a piece of sliced lemon on each fillet.
Drizzle with a little coconut water on each.
Now create a sealed parcel by joining together the paper ends and turning them several time to create a seal, try to allow a little room free above the fish and the seal.
Place the parcels on a oven baking tray and oven bake for 10 minutes.
Note: Allow fish to rest after cooking for 2 minutes, fish maybe served in the paper or opened and transferred to a serving plate.
10. Garnish with the ginger and snipped chives,

Tip: This fish meal will go well with steamed broccoli and or wilted spinach and steamed russet potatoes.

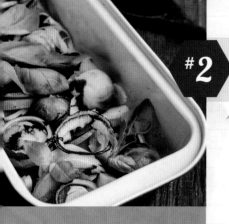

Root Veggie Casserole (Endo, Meso, Ecto)

Preparation Time: 15 minutes   *Cooking Time:* 30 minutes

What's in it

For the filing

2 parsnips, cut into ¼-inch rounds
2 carrots, cut into ¼-inch rounds
2 turnips cut into ¼ - inch rounds
2 cups brussel sprouts, halved
¾ cup vegetable broth
½ cup garlic cloves
1 bunch fresh asparagus, halved
½ cup eschallot bulbs
1 tsp chopped fresh thyme
¼ tsp ground black pepper
½ tsp coarse sea salt
1 tbsp balsamic vinager dressing
2 tbsp avocado oil
fresh basil leaves garnished

How to make it

Preheat oven to 350 F.
Combine all root vegetables, parsnips, carrots and turnips in a large bowl and mix in the avocado oil and salt and pepper.
Place in an 8x8-inch baking dish and pop into the oven, shake every 5 mins for 20 mins,
In a bowl, place the sprouts, eschallots and garlic, again sprinkle these with a little oil and lightly coat.
Add the sprout mixture to the partially baked root vegetables, continue cooking for an additional 15 minutes. Shaking occasionally to prevent overcooking/coloring.
Add the thyme and asparagus spears and continue to bake for another 5 mins.
Check that the vegetables are cooked and remove from the oven.
Portion out the roasted vegetables and sprinkle with a light drizzle of balsamic dressing and fresh basil leaves.

While root vegetables are particularly wonderful in the fall, you can take advantage of many of them all year long for this great casserole. Your body will love all of the fabulous nutrients it's receiving to help it stay fit and functioning at its best. While this dish is gluten-free, it certain isn't lacking in taste, pleasing even the pickiest of eaters while satisfying your dietary needs.

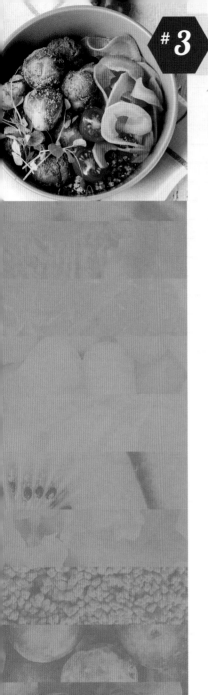

#3 Curried Brussels Sprouts
(Endo, Meso, Ecto)

Preparation Time: 20 minutes *Cooking Time:* 7-21 days fermentation

What's in it

13 oz brussels sprouts, outer leaves removed, trimmed and finely chopped
2 tsp sea salt
1/2 tsp cumin seeds
1/4 tsp yellow mustard seeds
1/4 tsp coriander seeds
1/3 cup freshly carrot juice
1 tsp mild curry powder
1/2 tsp ground turmeric
1 small green or purple cabbage leaf

Keynote: Requires 7-21 days of fermentation.

How to make it

Add brussels sprouts and 1 ½ tsp salt to a large bowl. Vigorously massage until they are soft and about ¼ cup of the liquid is released. Taste and add remaining ½ tsp salt, if needed. Cover and set aside.

Warm a dry skillet on medium-high. Add cumin, mustard and coriander seeds. Toast until they pop. About 3 to 5 minutes. Put spices in a grinder and grind to a powder.

Combine the spice mixture along with carrot juice, turmeric and curry to the sprouts. Use your hands (you might want to wear gloves) to massage the mixture into the sprouts.

Transfer brussels sprouts mixture and all juice to a 1-qt wide-mouth glass jar. Using your hand, press the mixture down firmly. This will release liquid and remove air pockets. Keep pressing until completely submerged.

Place a cabbage leaf in the jar on top of the sprout mixture. This will keep them submerged in the liquid. Seal the jar loosely with a lid.

Allow the mixture to ferment in a cool place away from direct sunlight, opening the jar once every 24 hours to release pressure. Press the cabbage down as needed to keep mixture submerged in liquid. Taste the mixture once in a while until it reaches a desired level of tanginess. About 7 to 21 days.

Once the desired level of tartness is reached, discard the cabbage leaf, seal the jar tightly and refrigerate for up to 3 months.

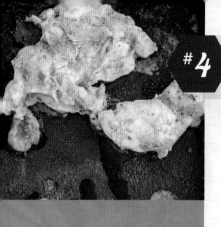

#4 Marinated Spiced Chicken (Meso, Endo)

Preparation Time: 10 minutes   *Cooking Time:* 20 minutes

What's in it

4 x 3 oz skinless boned out chicken thigh fillets
4 tsp avocado oil
½ cup of organic chicken stock

For the marinate

1 tsp turmeric
1 tsp crushed garlic
1/2 tsp Himalayan pink salt
1 tsp grated root ginger
2 eschallot bulbs, finely diced
1 tsp mild chopped chili
juice of 1 lime

How to make it

Prepare all marinate ingredients.
Place in a food blender and blend to a paste.
Rub equal amounts of the paste into each thigh.
Place thighs in a sealable lids container or zip lock bag
Add any remaining paste and store in the fridge for up to 24 hours.
Preheat oven to 300 ˚F.
Add some Avocado oil to a saute pan and warm.
Place the thigh's in the pan and very lightly seal on both side, immediatly transfer to a oven baking tray.
Warm the chicken stock and pour around the chicken.
Cover with foil or a pan lid and bake for 15 mins.

Dr Kareem Samhouri

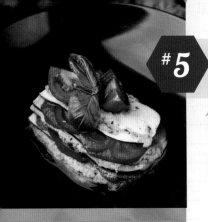

Zesty Zucchini Lasagna With Cashew Pesto (Endo, Meso, Ecto)

Preparation Time: 15 minutes   **Cooking Time:** 35 minutes

What's in it

1 ½ cups raw unsalted cashews

1 lemon, zested and juiced

12 large fresh basil leaves chopped, plus additional for garnish

¼ cup grated nutritional yeast

2 cloves garlic, chopped

3 zucchini, trimmed

pinch sea salt

1 ½ cups marinara sauce

2 roasted red bell peppers, sliced

2 tbsp water

How to make it

Preheat oven to 375 °F.

Soak cashews in a bowl of water for at least 4 hours, preferably overnight. Drain and put in food processor. To create pesto. Add lemon zest and juice, basil leaves, garlic, and 2 tbsp nutritional yeast. Pulse to break down the nuts. Add 1 to 2 tbsp water until the mixture becomes like ricotta cheese.

Slice the zucchini lengthwise into ½-inch planks using a mandoline. Place them on a baking sheet and sprinkle them with salt. After 10 minutes, blot the zucchini to remove excess salt and moisture.

Layer ¼ cup of marinara on the bottom of an 8-inch baking dish. Top with 2 layers of zucchini, one running top to bottom and one running crosswise. Spread half of the roasted bell pepper over the zucchini, and top with pesto. Spoon ½ cup marinara over the pesto and repeat the process.

Finish with 2 layers of zucchini and marinara. Sprinkle the rest of the nutritional yeast on top.

Cover and bake for 30 minutes.

Uncover and broil for 3 minutes until the top is browned.

Sprinkle basil on top.

It's not easy to find a delicious, gluten-free, vegan lasagna recipe, but this one satisfies all those requirements. Instead of meat, cheese and your typical lasagna noodles, it calls for fresh zucchini and raw cashews. Don't worry, you've still got those fabulous spices and marinara sauce that make it so delicious. In fact, it's so good, you may never go back to that old recipe.

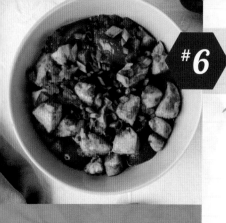

Chicken Chili (Meso, Ecto)

Preparation Time: 15 minutes   **Cooking Time:** 25 minutes

What's in it

2 tbsp coconut oil (warm)

1 small white onion, cut into 1/2-inch cubes

2 cloves garlic, peeled

1 jalapeno chile pepper, halved and seeded

1 ½ cups low-sodium chicken broth, divided

1 lb boneless, skinless chicken breast, cut into small chunks

2 tsp smoked paprika

1 tsp each ground cumin

1 tsp sea salt

½ tsp ground black pepper

1 small carrot, chopped finely

1 cup grape tomatoes, halved

chives for garnish

This chicken chili recipe is fantastic on a cold day. The chicken takes on all the wonderful flavors of the onion, garlic, jalapeno, paprika, and other spices. Plus, you get a good dose of vitamin A thanks to the addition of carrot. You can enjoy it as is, or with a bowl of savoury rice.

How to make it

Preheat oven to 400 ˚F.

Place onion and garlic on a pan and drizzle with coconut oil. Roast for 8 minutes and transfer to a blender or food processor.

Add jalapeno and ½ cup of broth. Puree.

Toss chicken with paprika, cumin, and salt and pepper in a bowl. Cook chicken in coconut oil, turn until brown, and transfer back to the bowl.

Heat 1 tsp coconut oil in chicken pan. Add carrots and cook until soft. Add remaining 1 cup broth and pureed vegetables. Bring to a simmer.

Put chicken back in pan and reduce heat to simmer for 10 minutes.

Add tomatoes, simmer until they are soft and chicken is fully cooked through. About 7 minutes.

Garnish with chives.

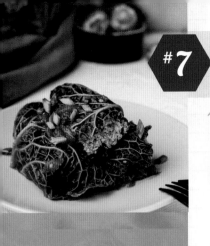

Cabbage Roll Ups (Endo, Meso, Ecto)

Preparation Time: 15 minutes   *Cooking Time:* 20 minutes

What's in it

1 large head green or savoy cabbage
2 tbsp coconut oil
1/2 yellow onion, diced
1 carrot, diced
1 rib celery, diced
2 cups cremini mushrooms, diced
1 tsp caraway seeds
2 tbsp yellow miso
2 tbsp ground flaxseeds
½ tsp ground black pepper
½ cup finely chopped unsalted walnuts
3 cups tricolor quinoa, cooked
2 tbsp finely chopped fresh chives, plus additional for serving
1 ½ cups organic marinara sauce

How to make it

Place a whole cabbage in water. Cover and cook for 3 minutes. Drain off the water and remove 8 outer leaves. Cut and save the remaining cabbage for another dish.
Warm coconut oil in a pan on medium heat. Add onion, carrot, and celery and cook for 5 minutes.
Add mushrooms and caraway seeds. Stir constantly and cook for 3 more minutes. Put mixture in a food processor and add miso, flaxseeds and pepper. Finely chop the mixture while keeping texture. Add the walnuts and pulse to blend. Transfer everything to a large bowl and add quinoa and chives.
Make rolls by laying cabbage leaves on a flat surface. Fill a cup ½ way full of quinoa mixture and place near the stem end of the leaf. Press the mixture into an oval about half the length of the leaf. Fold the top of the leaf down toward the stem then fold the 2 sides over the filling and roll up. Repeat with the rest of the leaves.
Pour half of the marinara sauce into a shallow pot. Spread sauce to coat the bottom. Place the cabbage rolls, folded side down, into the pan. Pour the remaining sauce over the rolls.
Put a lid on the pot and cook on medium-low for 10 minutes.
Garnish with chives.

Cabbage makes a great base for so many dishes, and in this case, it serves as the "roll." These roll-ups are stuffed with tasty flavors and nutrition, with lots of protein thanks to the quinoa and walnuts. It's a great healthy dish to bring to a potluck or serve at a dinner party, satisfying just about every taste and dietary need.

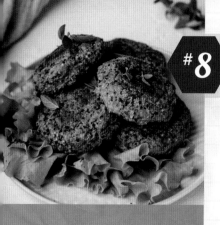

#8 Quinoa Cakes (Meso, Ecto)

Preparation Time: 15 minutes   *Cooking Time:* 20 minutes

These cakes are nutritious and filling enough for a complete meal. They're gluten-free and loaded with essential nutrients, thanks to ingredients like sweet potato, kale and tomatoes. With the quinoa, you'll be getting a hefty dose of protein and all nine amino acids.

What's in it

- 1 ½ cups quinoa, cooked
- 2 tbsp ground flax, plus 6 tbsp water
- 1 cup kale, de-stemmed and chopped
- ½ cup rolled oats, ground into flour
- ½ cup sweet potato, finely grated
- ¼ cup sun dried tomatoes, finely chopped in oil
- ¼ cup sunflower seeds
- ¼ cup basil leaves, chopped fine
- 2 tbsp onion, finely diced
- 1 clove garlic, minced
- 1 tbsp tahini paste
- 1 ½ tsp dried oregano
- 1 ½ tsp red vinegar
- ½ tsp salt
- red pepper flakes to taste

How to make it

Preheat oven to 400 ˚F. Line baking sheet with parchment paper.

Combine flax and water in a small bowl and set aside for 5 minutes to thicken.

Mix all ingredients together in a large bowl along with 1 ½ cups cooked quinoa. Stir until the mixture binds together.

Form the mixture into ¼ cup patties using your hands. Be sure to pack tightly so that they stay together. Place on a baking sheet.

Bake for 15 minutes, then flip and bake for 10 more minutes until brown and firm.

Cool for 5 minutes.

Serve with large side salad.

The Busy Cookbook | *Dr Kareem Samhouri*

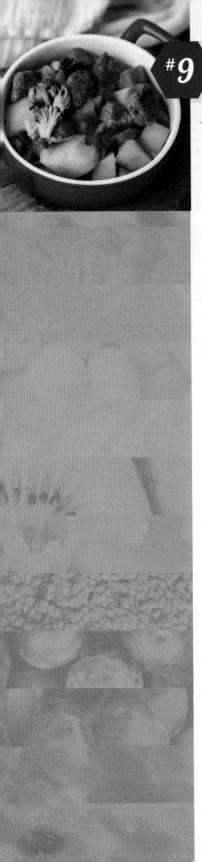

#9 Braised Beef or Lamb Spring Casserole (Meso, Ecto)

Preparation Time: 15 minutes   *Cooking Time:* 120-150 minutes

What's in it

10oz lean diced braising beef or lamb

3 tbsp rice bran oil

1 cup diced carrot

2 cups diced russet potatoes

½ cup peeled whole garlic

½ cup peeled whole eschallots

1 cup diced butternut squash

1 1/4 cup peeled and diced plum tomatoes

2 cups organic beef broth

1 bunch broccolini

¼ tsp dried oregano

3 bay leaves

Himalayan sea salt to taste

1 tsp ghee butter

How to make it

Preheat oven to 350 ˚F.

Add oil to pan and seal the red meat and set aside in a strainer to allow the excess liquids to drain.

In a lidable braising pan, add the strained liquid along with the carrots, lightly cook for a few minutes, then return the red meat to the pan.

Add salt, bay leaves, tomatoes and beef broth.

Cover with lid and braise for 1 hour.

Add the potatoes, eschallots and garlic bulbs and return to braise for 40 minutes.

Add the butternut squash and dried oregano, continue to braise.

Braise until meat is tender, check seasoning,

Serve in large bowls and top with cooked broccolini sauteed in ghee.

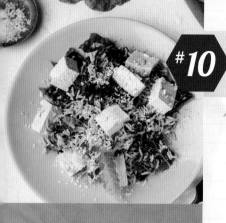

Kale and Coconut Tofu Salad (Meso, Ecto)

#10

🍴 *Preparation Time:* 10 minutes   ♨ **Cooking Time:** 25 minutes

What's in it

A salad that checks all the boxes: vegan, gluten-free, and packed with nutrition and flavor. It's the perfect blend of slightly sweet and slightly salty to satisfy those taste buds while taking advantage of the superfood power of kale. The brown rice and tofu both add protein to prevent hunger pangs in the night.

1 cup short grain brown rice, cooked
sea salt to taste
⅓ cup olive oil
1 tsp toasted sesame oil
2 tbsp liquid aminos
1 ½ lbs kale, de-stemmed, ribs removed, and chopped
½ cup unsweetened coconut flakes
½ lb extra firm tofu, cut into 1/4 -inch cubes

How to make it

Preheat oven to 350 ° F. Put racks in the lower and upper thirds of the oven.
Whisk the olive oil, sesame oil and aminos together to make dressing.
Place kale, tofu, and coconut in a large bowl. Drizzle two-thirds of the dressing on the kale and toss.
Spread the kale out on 2 rimmed baking sheets and bake for 25 minutes, until crispy.
Stir a couple of times during baking and shift the pans halfway through.
Put the mixture back in a bowl and toss with the remaining dressing and rice.
Season with salt and serve immediately.

Dr Kareem Samhouri

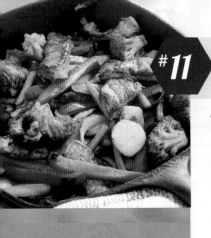

#11

Steak and Veggie Stir Fry
(Meso, Ecto)

Preparation Time: 15 minutes   *Cooking Time:* 10 minutes

What's in it

For the sauce
- 2 tbsp coconut aminos
- 2 tbsp warm water
- 2 garlic cloves, minced
- ½ tsp fresh ginger, grated

For the main dish
- 1 lb steak, sliced into ¼ inch thick strips
- 2 tbsp coconut oil
- 1 cup broccoli, chopped
- 1 cup red onion, cut in strips
- 1 cup green beans, trimmed
- 1 cup finely sliced carrots
- 1 cup red bell pepper, cut in strips
- 1 tbsp sesame seeds
- 3 tbsp green onion, chopped
- ¼ cup water chestnuts, sliced

Stir-fry is such a great way to sneak lots of vegetables into your diet. Plus, it's super easy to put together. This one includes a fantastic mix of broccoli, green beans, onions, and peppers to help ensure you meet your daily nutritional needs. With the addition of steak, you'll satisfy your meat craving and get plenty of protein and iron.

How to make it

Warm wok over medium heat and add coconut oil.
Add steak to the skillet and let brown on all sides.
Remove from heat and set aside.
Add sliced onion, broccoli, green beans, carrots and red peppers. Saute for 5 minutes.
Combine aminos, warm water, minced garlic and grated ginger in a small bowl and whisk.
Combine meat and sauce in the pan with vegetables, toss and heat through, about 2 minutes.
Top stir fry with sliced water chestnuts, chopped green onions, and sesame seeds.

Tip: Ectomorphs - cook the vegetebale until your desired doneness, then add the beef. Add a portion of Rice

.

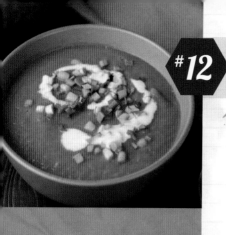

Easy Pumpkin and Carrot Soup (Endo, Meso, Ecto)

Preparation Time: 10 minutes   *Cooking Time:* 35 minutes

Though one of our favorites in the fall, this soup can still be enjoyed all year long. Thanks to the pumpkin pie spice flavor combined with onion and broth, this savory dish brings back memories of Thanksgiving.

What's in it

- 1 medium onion, grated
- 2 tbsp avocado oil
- 1 29-oz can pure pumpkin
- 2 cups sliced carrots
- 2 cups carrot juice
- ½ cup almond milk
- 4 cups organic vegetable stock
- pink or black Himalayan salt to taste
- 1 cup diced steamed fennel
- 1 cup diced steamed butternut squash
- ¼ cup snipped shallots or chives

How to make it

Warm oil in a saucepan over medium-high heat. Add the onion and cook. Stirring 2 minutes or until soft.

Stir in the squash, carrots, carrot juice, vegetable broth and salt.

Return the liquid to a simmer and cook for 30 minutes, stirring occasionally.

Once the carrots are cooked, place the liquid in a blender no more than half full at a time and blend until smooth, add a little almond milk to correct the consistency.

Place the warm fennel and squash in bowls and pour over the soup.

Garnish with the snipped shallots or chives.

Dr Kareem Samhouri

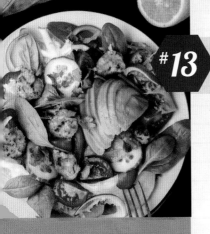

#13 Shrimp Salad with Avocado (Meso)

Preparation Time: 10 minutes *Cooking Time:* 10 minutes

What's in it

- 1 lb medium shrimp
- 1 tsp cajun spice
- 2 cloves garlic, pressed and grated
- pinch of sea salt
- 2 tbsp ghee butter

For the salad

- 4 cups romaine lettuce, chopped
- 2 cups baby spinach leaves
- 3 medium roma tomatoes, sliced
- ½ medium red onion, sliced thin
- ½ english cucumber, sliced
- 2 avocados, peeled, pitted, and sliced
- ½ cup diced mixed bell peppers, 1 inch pieces

For the dressing

- 3 tbsp lemon juice
- ½ cup cilantro, finely chopped
- 3 tbsp extra virgin olive oil
- 1 tsp sea salt
- ½ tsp black pepper

This recipe is a great way to use up some of your garden's bounty. Enjoy this on a warm summer's day at a picnic, or any time of the year.

How to make it

Pat shrimp dry with paper towels and place in a medium bowl.

Add 1 tsp cajun spice, 2 pressed garlic cloves, and a pinch of salt. Stir to mix.

Heat a large non-stick pan over medium-heat. Add 2 tablespoons butter. Once melted, add shrimp in a single layer. Saute for 2 minutes per side or until cooked through. Transfer to a plate and set aside.

Combine lettuce and spinach and place on 3 plates. Top with onion, tomato, cucumber, avocado, peppers and shrimp.

Combine 3 tablespoons fresh lemon juice with ½ cup cilantro and stir. Add 3 tablespoons olive oil and season with salt and pepper.

Drizzle over salad and serve immediately.

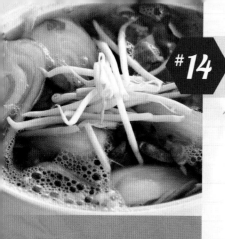

#14 Asian Style Broth (Endo, Meso, Ecto)

Preparation Time: 10 minutes   *Cooking Time:* 15 minutes

What's in it

- 8 1/2 cup organic vegetable broth / stock
- 1 cup sliced bok choy
- ½ cup sliced bamboo shoot
- ½ sliced water chestnuts
- 1 cup mung bean sprouts
- 1 cup quartered artichoke hearts
- 1 cup finely sliced napa cabbage
- ½ tsp chili flakes
- ½ cup finely sliced carrots

Garnish

- 2 sheets of broken up Nori seaweed
- fresh cilantro leaves
- picked pink sushi ginger
- snipped chives

How to make it

In a medium soup pan, warm through the broth.
Add the carrots and allow to simmer for 2 minutes.
Add the bok choy and cabbage, simmer for 3 minutes.
Add the bamboo, water chestnuts, mung sprouts, artichokes and chili flakes.
Simmer for 4 minutes.
In serving bowls place the seaweed piece in first, ladle over the broth and with a spoon stir the seaweed into the broth.
Garnish with the sushi ginger, cilantro and chives.

Tip: Ectomorph, you can add some cooked warm purple rice into the broth.

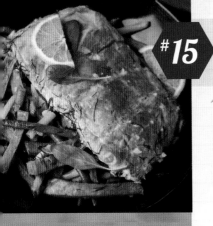

Salmon and Veggie Pan (Meso, Endo)

/ **Preparation Time:** 10 minutes   **Cooking Time:** 30 minutes

What's in it

For the dressing

- 2 tbsp avocado oil
- 1 lemon, juiced
- 1 garlic clove, minced

For the fish

- 1 ¼ wild-caught salmon fillet, cut into 4 portions
- 1 medium sweet potato, peeled and sliced thinly
- 12 oz green beans, trimmed
- ½ small red onion, slice thinly
- 1 tbsp fresh dill
- sea salt to taste
- black pepper to taste
- ½ lemon, sliced thinly
- parchment paper

Wild-caught salmon is one of the best sources of healthy fatty acids and protein, but after a while, that same old piece of wild-caught salmon with a side salad gets a little boring. This recipe spices things up while making great use of our ocean's bounty. The added vegetables help meet your vitamin and mineral needs, while adding to the rich flavor.

How to make it

Dressing

Whisk all ingredients together in a small bowl.

Fish

Preheat oven to 425 °F.

Place parchment paper on a large rimmed baking sheet.

Put sweet potatoes on the baking sheet. Add green beans and red onions.

Drizzle half the dressing over the vegetables. Toss.

Place salmon filets between the vegetables.

Top with remaining dressing.

Place lemon slices on top of each filet. Sprinkle dill, sea salt, and pepper on top.

Bake for 20 minutes or until salmon flakes easily with a fork.

Remove filets and cover with a plate. Return vegetables to oven and cook 10 more minutes until potatoes are tender.

Remove from pan and serve salmon on top of vegetebles. Add sea salt and pepper and additional lemon slices.

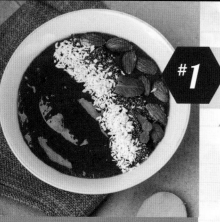

#1 Chocolate Banana Bowl (Endo, Meso, Ecto)

🍴 *Preparation Time:* 5 minutes   🍲 *Cooking Time:* 3 minutes

What's in it

1 frozen banana
½ cup blueberries
1 handful spinach
2 tbsp almond butter
1 tbsp raw cacao powder
½ tsp pure vanilla extract
½ cup almond milk
1 tsp raw honey

For topping

raw coconut, shredded
chia seeds
crushed almonds

How to make it

Place all ingredients in a blender and mix well.
Top with chopped almonds, shredded raw coconut
and chia seeds as desired.

Yes, you can enjoy the rich and delicious taste of chocolate, even for breakfast! This smoothie bowl contains bananas that are rich in potassium and magnesium, and antioxidant-rich berries and greens. Add a scoop of hemp protein powder for an extra boost.

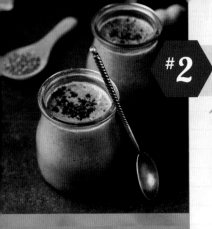

#2 *Creamy Cocoa Pudding*

Preparation Time: 5 minutes   *Cooking Time:* 15 minutes

What's in it

½ cup chia seeds
1 cup almond milk
1 tbsp organic raw cacao powder
2 tsp raw honey
2 tsp organic bee pollen

How to make it

Mix the chia seeds with the almond milk, honey and cacao powder. Set aside for 15 minutes.
Serve in small glasses and garnish with bee pollen.

If you like chocolate, you are going to love the rich taste of this cocoa pudding. The health benefits of raw cocoa include its ability to boost not only your energy levels but also your mood. Cocoa in its raw form also contains twenty times more antioxidant power than blueberries.

SOUPS:

Here are a couple bonus soup recipes that are absolutely delicious and appropriate for all body types: endomorphs, mesomorphs, and ectomoprhs.

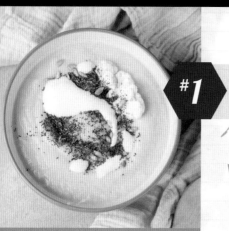

 # 1

Cauliflower Nut Soup

Preparation Time: 5 minutes   *Cooking Time:* 20 minutes

What's in it

> 1 ½ tbsp olive oil
> 1 medium onion, chopped
> 2 garlic cloves, grated
> ½ tsp salt
> ½ tsp pepper
> 1 cauliflower head, cut into florets
> 4 cups vegetable broth

Suggested toppings

> 1 cup plain Greek yogurt
> 1 tbsp dried mint
> 2 tbsp toasted pine nuts

How to make it

> Put oil in a pan and heat. Add onion, garlic, salt and pepper and saute over medium heat until translucent.
> Add cauliflower and cook for about a minute.
> Add in vegetable broth and bring to a boil.
> Reduce the heat to low and simmer with a lid on for about 15 minutes.
> Remove from the heat and use a hand blender to blend well.
> Top with yogurt, mint and nuts.

This creamy soup contains B vitamins riboflavin, niacin and thiamine. It is bursting with a robust flavor that will make you forget you are on a detox. The dietary fiber in this soup will keep your digestive system functioning smoothly and the vitamin C is important for immune health.

My Body Transform | Dr Kareem Samhouri

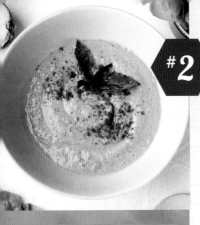

#2 Cold Cucumber and Avocado Soup

Preparation Time: 5 minutes　　*Cooking Time:* 3 minutes

What's in it

1 large cucumber, peeled and deseeded

1 tbsp fresh onion, minced

1 medium avocado, peeled

1 tbsp olive oil

1 tbsp lemon juice

1 tbsp apple cider vinegar

1 cup filtered water

¼ tsp sea salt

¼ tsp chili powder

dash cayenne pepper

paprika for garnish

How to make it

Put all ingredients in a blender and blend until smooth. Garnish with extra cucumber and paprika, if desired.

Cucumbers are rich in vitamins B, potassium, and magnesium and also contain a great deal of water which makes them a great addition to any detox diet. Avocados add just the right amount of healthy fat to balance out this delicious whole-food soup.

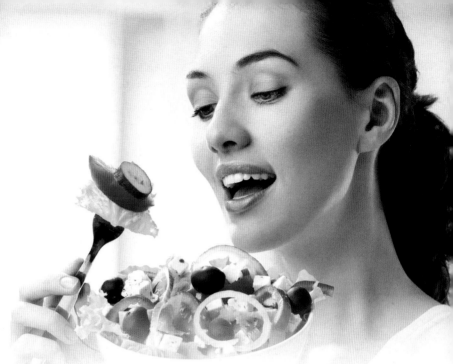

CONCLUSION:

It is our sincere hope and desire that you have experienced a radical shift in your eating habits, health, and body image in a rather short period of time. By learning how to clean out your body, transition back to a healthy diet, and then eat for your body, in specific, you are giving yourself a gift that keeps on giving. Plus, you are setting an example for everyone you love, so they too can care for themselves in a personalized and logical way.

You see, it's super simple to eat well if you follow a plan for a little while, play with recipes and adjust them to your palette, and learn which foods pair best with your body, at which times. Sounds like a lot at first, although this is a very intuitive process:

> *Look at, think of, or hold food.*
>
> *Ask yourself how you'll feel after you eat it.*

Notice how you feel inside your body after asking this question, or if you hear any internal dialogue, or if you see or sense something out of nowhere.

Listen to your intuition and see how it went. Did you choose a recipe that agreed with you? How did you feel? How did you feel the last time you ate the meal? What was the same or different?

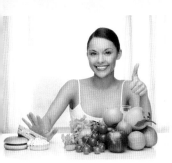

Learn which foods -- and which specific ingredients -- feel the best inside of your body and give you the cleanest energy. Then, choose more of those foods and expand upon your palette slowly. Notice the likelihood that foods that work well for you are also in the same body shape category as you. Then, take note of other people with your body shape/size, and how they eat. Are they healthier or less healthy than you? And how closely do they eat compared to what you've just discovered about you? I suspect you'll be surprised how much of a difference it makes to know how to eat for your body, in specific.

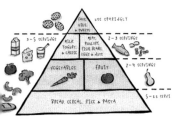

And this is the final point: please have grace with yourself and others. We were all educated with the Food Guide Pyramid, calories in vs out, and macronutrient ratios (carbs, fats, and proteins). The idea of each of us eating uniquely for our own bodies is a lot for a family to wrap their heads around at first. It makes sense and works quickly, and many recipes can be shared by everyone in your family during otherwise stable circumstances. However, specific customizations may need to take place, like meat on the side, or no gluten, or adjusting a meal completely for someone who is going through a moment of emotional distress.

Once you are able to understand the differences in natural eating patterns between you and your family members, you can layer in the emotional impact of eating and the conversations that surround meal-time. You may find that the most stimulating conversation for some people is a source of stress and digestive disrupt in others. Simply observe for now, recognize you are unique, the goal of eating is to gain energy and health. So, we must learn what is healthy eating, and when we can eat certain foods that match our bodies.

One thing is for sure: We believe in you.

YOU CAN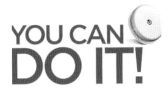
DO IT!

In support of you reaching your full health potential,

The Create My Workout Nutrition Team CMW
https://CreateMyWorkout.com